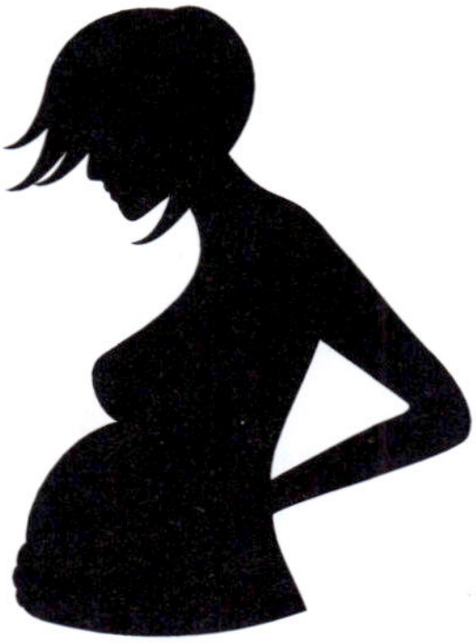

# OBSTETRICS AND GYNAECOLOGY ST1
## INTERVIEW BOOK

SECOND EDITION

OBSTETRICS AND GYNAECOLOGY ST1
INTERVIEW BOOK

# OBSTETRICS AND GYNAECOLOGY ST1
## INTERVIEW BOOK

SECOND EDITION

**Dr Neha Shah MBBS MRCOG**
Specialty Trainee in Obstetrics and Gynaecology
London Deanery

**Dr Noshali Wimalaweera MBBS BSC**
Specialty Trainee in Obstetrics and Gynaecology
London Deanery

**Dr Chawan Baran MBBS MRCOG**
Specialty Trainee in Obstetrics and Gynaecology
Kent Surrey Sussex Deanery

OBSTETRICS AND GYNAECOLOGY ST1
INTERVIEW BOOK

Obstetrics and Gynaecology ST1 Interview Book is affiliated with the Obstetrics and Gynaecology ST1 Interview Course (obsandgynae.net).



**ISBN 9781675766576**

OBSTETRICS AND
GYNAECOLOGY ST1
INTERVIEW BOOK

# PREFACE

The **Nepalese Doctors Association UK** (NDAUK) is one of the most prestigious organisations that has maintained the highest standards of professional integrity right from its inception in 1985, and has become a symbol of unity among doctors of Nepalese origin. We have on going inspiring projects to raise charity funds to help post earthquake reconstruction and rehabilitation in Nepal.

I am delighted to present the second edition of this interview book to you, written by Dr Neha Shah, Dr Noshali Wimalaweera and Dr Chawan Baran. The book provides a valuable resource for any doctor applying for Obstetric and Gynaecology specialty training. The charity fund raised by this project will go directly to buy more ambulances to transport sick and vulnerable patients in the remote eastern region of Taplejung, Nepal. For the first time in the history of NDA UK, we are dedicating a special preface in a book to acknowledge a significant contribution made by the authors.

**MISS BEENA SUBBA**
*Consultant Obstetrician & Gynaecologist*
*MD, FRCOG*
**Chair, NDAUK**

# ABOUT THE AUTHORS

**Neha Shah** is a specialty trainee in the North Central and East London Deanery having obtained her training post in 2015. Neha had created a large quantity of notes in preparation for her ST1 interviews and, after securing a place in one of the most competitive rotations in the country, wanted to use her knowledge and experience to help other budding trainees. Neha and her colleague Chawan launched the *Obstetrics and Gynaecology ST1 Interview Course* in 2015. The following year they went on to publish the first edition of this *Obstetrics and Gynaecology ST1 Interview Book.*

Neha, with her colleague Noshali, have created this second edition of the book, refining and updating it to cover the change from a regional to national interview process.

**Chawan Baran** is a specialty trainee in the Kent Surrey Sussex Deanery having obtained her training post in 2015. Chawan worked with Neha to launch the *Obstetrics and Gynaecology ST1 Interview Course* and went on to contribute to the first edition of this interview book.

**Noshali Wimalaweera** is a specialty trainee in the North Central and East London Deanery having obtained her training post in 2019. With her recent experience of the interviews, Noshali has been a valuable contributor to this second edition and has helped refine the interview book to make it more relevant to current interviews.

Whilst there have been significant changes in this second edition, the authors would like to extend a note of gratitude to **Minhui Wong**, a specialty trainee in the North Central and East London Deanery, who edited the first edition of Obstetrics and Gynaecology ST1 Interview Book.

# OBSTETRICS AND GYNAECOLOGY ST1 INTERVIEW BOOK

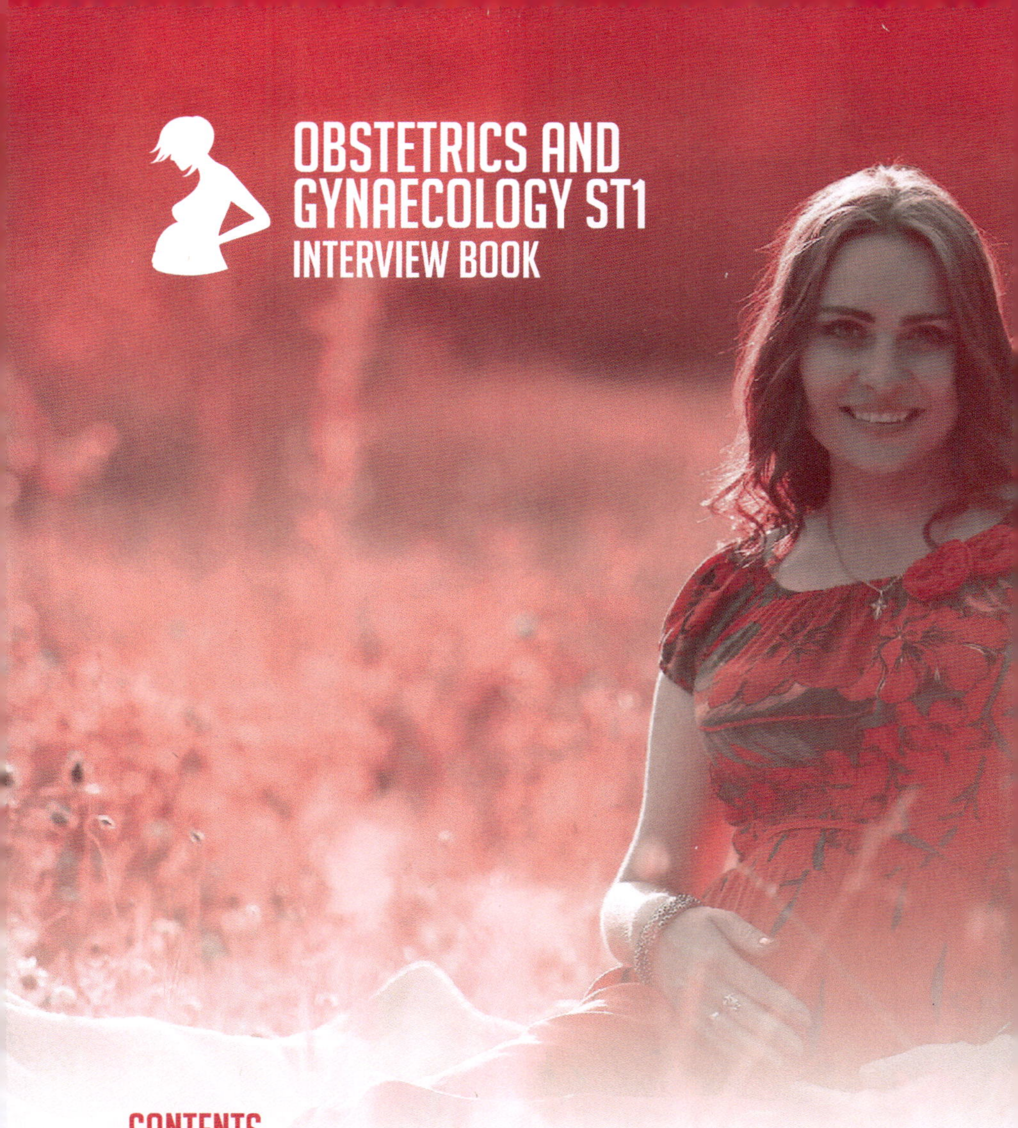

## CONTENTS

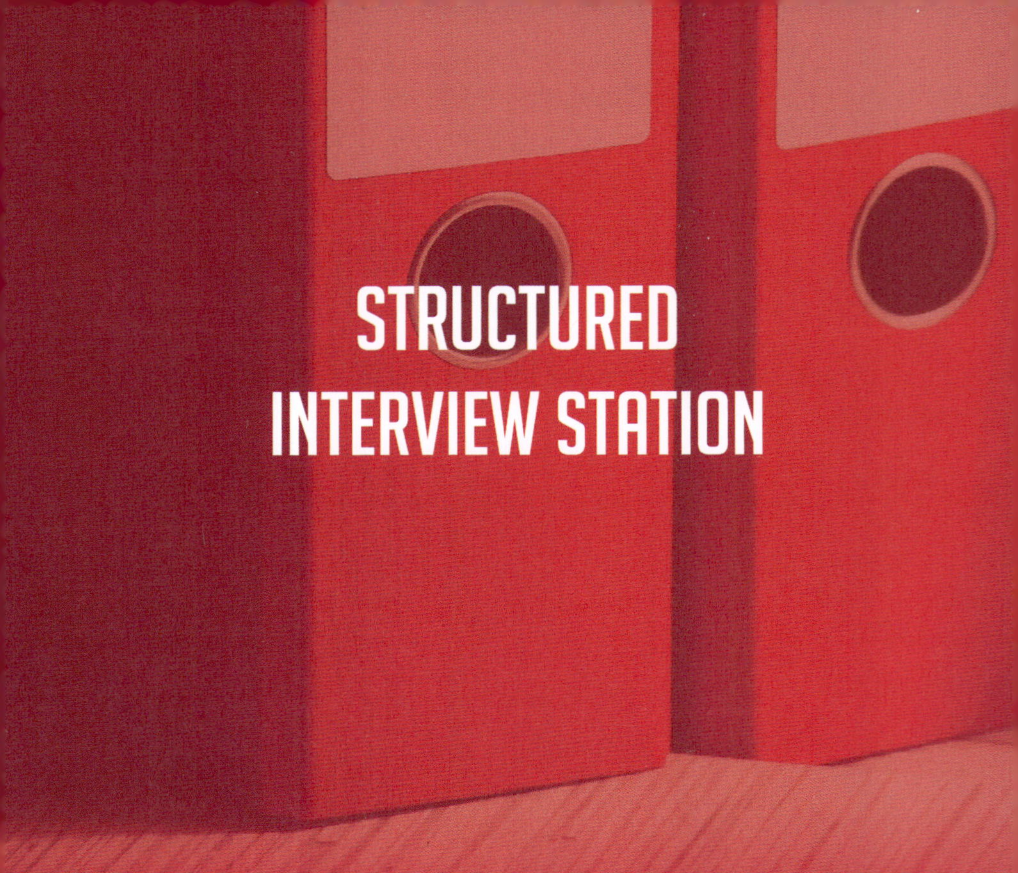

# STRUCTURED INTERVIEW STATION

OBSTETRICS AND GYNAECOLOGY ST1 INTERVIEW BOOK

obsandgynae.net

# STRUCTURED INTERVIEW STATION

Structured interview stations commonly cover four themes, which carry approximately equal weighting.

- Understanding of and commitment to the specialty
- Experience outside obstetrics and gynaecology, leadership and team-working
- Quality improvement measures (including audit)
- Teaching and research

Interviewers are trying to ascertain your insight into the specialty, therefore it is important to speak to existing trainees, read the person specification and go through the RCOG website.

Each station is only about ten minutes long so there is not a lot of time to highlight your strengths. As such, it is imperative to be concise and time your answers appropriately. We recommend not spending more than one minute per answer, and to split your time equally between the above categories.

# WHY OBSTETRICS AND GYNAECOLOGY?

This will probably be the first question you will be asked, so it is vital to have a specific and personalised answer to give yourself a good starting impression.

Example reasons:

- A diverse specialty encompassing acute management (e.g. labour ward), chronic management (e.g. gynaecology clinics), diagnostics of ultrasound and surgical management.
- Strong communication aspect.
- Surgical specialty.
- Diagnostics of ultrasound.
- Ability to make a significant difference to women's quality of life.
- Physiology of pregnancy fascinating.
- Multidisciplinary team approach.

# WHAT WOULD YOUR TRAINING PRIORITIES BE IN THE FIRST 12 MONTHS?

- Achieve progress appropriate to ST1/ST2 in the 14 CiP (Capabilities in Practice) and other requirements to pass ARCP
- Focus on obtaining labour ward experience.
- Pass MRCOG part 1.
- Develop basic ultrasound competencies (and attend an ultrasound course).
- By doing the above, develop the skills to be competent when second on call (ST3).

# THE STRUCTURE OF THE TRAINING PROGRAMME

Obstetrics and Gynaecology is a 7 year run-through training programme, ranging from ST1 through to ST7.

The Obstetrics and Gynaecology curriculum was changed in 2019. The reason for the change in the curriculum was to support a move away from a 'disease-based' structure to encourage a more "patient-centered" approach that prioritises the needs and complexities of each individual patient.

# THE NEW CURRICULUM (2019)

The new core curriculum consists of **4 Professional Identities** (PIs):

- Professional Identity 1: Healthcare Professional
- Professional Identity 2: Researcher, Scholar and Educator
- Professional Identity 3: Clinical Expert
- Professional Identity 4: Champion for Women's Health.

Each PI consists of a number of **Capabilities in Practice** (CiPs), which are high-level statements setting out what a doctor should be able to do at the end of training. There are a total of 14 CiPs which are listed in the table below.

| **DEVELOPING THE DOCTOR (GENERIC)** | |
|---|---|
| **Professional identity 1: Healthcare professional** | |
| CiP 1 | The doctor is able to apply medical knowledge, clinical skills and professional values for the provision of high-quality and safe patient-centered care |
| CiP 2 | The doctor is able to successfully work within health organisations |
| CiP 3 | The doctor is a leader who has vision, engages and delivers results |
| CiP 4 | The doctor is able to design and implement quality improvement projects or interventions |
| CiP 5 | The doctor understands and applies basic Human Factors principles and practice at individual, team, organisational and system levels |

| Professional identity 2: Researcher, scholar and educator | |
|---|---|
| CiP 6 | The doctor takes an active role in helping others to develop themselves |
| CiP 7 | The doctor is able to engage with research and promote innovation |
| CiP 8 | The doctor is effective as a teacher and supervisor of healthcare professionals |
| **Developing the Obstetrician & Gynaecologist (specialty-specific)** | |
| Professional identity 3: Clinical expert | |
| CiP 9 | The doctor is competent in recognising, assessing and managing emergencies in gynaecology and early pregnancy |
| CiP 10 | The doctor is competent in recognising, assessing and managing emergencies in obstetrics |
| CiP 11 | The doctor is competent in recognising, assessing and managing non-emergency gynaecology and early pregnancy care |
| CiP 12 | The doctor is competent in recognising, assessing and managing non-emergency obstetrics care |
| Professional identity 4: Champion for women's health | |
| CiP 13 | The doctor is able to champion the healthcare needs of people from all groups within society. |
| CiP 14 | The doctor takes an active role in implementing public health priorities for women and works within local, national and international structures to promote health and prevent disease. |

Each CiP is supported by the key skills expected to be demonstrated by a CCT holder.

**Example:**

| **CiP 4: The doctor is able to design and implement quality improvement projects or interventions.** | |
|---|---|
| **Key Skills** | **Descriptors** |
| Understands quality improvement (quality is safety, experience and efficacy) | Understands the difference between quality improvement and research.<br>• Understands QI methodology such as Plan, Do, Study, Act cycles (PDSA).<br>• Understands the concepts of big data and national clinical audit.<br>• Appreciates the importance of stakeholders in QI work encouraging involvement with patient groups e.g. Maternity Voices Partnership. |
| Undertakes and evaluates impact of QI interventions | Is actively involved in QI initiatives (examples include: clinical audit, guideline development, implementation of national guidance, service improvement).<br>• Considers the best way to share learning.<br>• Evaluates quality improvement projects and how these can work at a local, regional and national level. |

In the final two years of training, Trainee doctors still have to complete **two Advanced Training Skills Modules** (ATSMs) OR **one subspecialty programme** to be eligible for **Completion of Core Training** (CCT).

# ST1/ST2 COMPETENCIES

### Procedures (OSATS - Objective Structured Assessment of Technical Skills)

- Cervical smear
- Basic caesarean section
- Non-rotational assisted vaginal delivery
- Surgical management of miscarriage
- Manual removal of placenta
- Perineal repair
- Endometrial biopsy
- Insertion of IUS or IUCD

### Courses

- Basic Practical Skills in Obstetrics and Gynaecology
- CTG Training
- Obstetric Simulation Course (e.g. PROMPT, ALSO)
- Basic ultrasound course
- Third degree tear course
- Resilience Course (e.g. STEP-UP)

### Workplace Based Assessments

- Mini CEXs (Mini Clinical Evaluation Exercise)
- CBDs (Case Based Discussions)
- Reflective practices
- NOTSS (Non-Technical Skills for Surgeons)

### Examinations

- MRCOG part 1

### Teaching attendance

- 100% of available regional teaching

### Other

- TO2s (Team observation) to be completed atleast twice a year
- One completed and presented clinical governance project per year

# REQUIREMENTS OF ST1

## NOTES :

- Formative OSATs– shows evidence of training since last ARCP. Optional but encouraged.
- Summative OSATs– Shows competence (Need at least 3 by at least two difference assessors)least two difference assessors).

A recent change in the training pathway :

- There is a greater emphasis on ultrasound, with ultrasound competencies and attendance at a basic ultrasound course now being a requirement of ST1 and ST2.

# THE FUTURE OF OBSTETRICS AND GYNAECOLOGY

- Shift towards 24-hour consultant-delivered care (versus consultant-led care).
- Centralisation of specialist services – e.g. endometriosis centres.
- Shift of workload to community – e.g. community gynaecology.
- Trend towards medical management of gynaecological conditions and therefore a reduction in surgical management (e.g. heavy menstrual bleeding was previously often managed by hysterectomy. Now there are a number of alternative medical options including mirena coil and endometrial ablation).
- Increase in the number of female trainees in the workforce – increase in part-time workers and maternity leave.
- Increasing maternal age at childbirth, thereby increasing co-morbidities in the obstetric population with a greater need to manage medical conditions in obstetrics.

**TOP TIP:**

When mentioning the shift towards 24-hour consultant delivered services, state that you understand this means as a consultant you may be working a shift pattern (including night shifts on-site) and you are willing to do so because:

1. Patient safety is your priority.
2. Although you will be working night shifts, you understand that you will be given compensatory time off.

**TOP TIP:**

When discussing the increase in co-morbidities in the obstetric population and the increasing emphasis on management of medical conditions in pregnancy, mention that this is highlighted by the MBRRACE report. The MBRRACE Maternal Mortality report 2017 shows that INDIRECT causes (deaths due to pre-existing medical conditions or mental health problems) continue to be the leading cause for maternal mortality, accounting for 56% of deaths in the 2013-2015 trienium.

On a positive note, there has been a significant 23% decrease in indirect maternal mortality since 2010–12 primarily due to a decrease in deaths from sepsis and influenza. Cardiac disease remains the leading cause of indirect maternal death during or up to six weeks after the end of pregnancy

# CHALLENGES FACING TRAINEES AND HOW TO OVERCOME THEM

| Challenge | How to overcome |
| --- | --- |
| Insufficient training opportunities (secondary to European Working Time Directive and reduced surgical workload) | Maximise training opportunities- workplace based assessments (WBA), eLearning, courses, simulation training, additional reading. |
| Fragmentation of care (secondary to European Working Time Directive) | Meticulous hand-over, be proactive in following up cases |
| Increased litigation | Accurate documentation, seek senior support when required, good communication skills |

## NOTES :

- Workplace Based Assessments include
- Case Based Discussions (CBDs)
- Clinical Evaluation Exercises (Mini-CEX)
- Objective Structured Assessment of Technical Skills (OSATs)
- Non-Technical Skills for Surgeons (NOTSS)

# TELL US ABOUT YOUR TEACHING EXPERIENCE

- Use a maximum of three examples, covering a range of teaching styles (e.g. small group/large group, didactic/interactive, formal/informal,
- Clinical/communication/practical skills).
- Discuss feedback received.
- Mention if you have had any formal teaching experience.
- When describing feedback
  - First mention positive feedback.
  - Then mention any negative feedback.
  - Finish by explaining how you have used that negative feedback to improve your teaching practice, thereby finishing on a positive note.

Examples of Positive Feedback

1) Clear and concise
2) Positive and encouraging
3) Sets appropriate goals
4) Involves students
5) Able to adapt to students level of knowledge
7) Interactive teaching style

Examples of Positive Feedback

1) Did not provide clear objectives at the start of the session and ensure these had been reached at the end. In future teaching sessions, I have implemented this and found that not only did feedback from students improve, but it gave me an objective measure of my teaching skills.

2) Slides "too wordy". I now limit myself to a maximum number of words per slide and aim that 50% of the information I present is not directly written on slides.

3) Did not involve the quieter members of the group. Although I lead very interactive teaching sessions, only certain students would actively answer questions and discuss cases. I have now changed my practice so that I ask students to discuss questions or cases in groups to ensure that they are all involved without too much pressure on individual students.

# HOW DO YOU KNOW THAT YOU ARE A GOOD TEACHER?

- Positive feedback (see page 9).
- Objective measures of your teaching – students passing exams, or an objective test at the end of teaching sessions.
- Improvement in clinical practice (e.g. teaching on postpartum haemorrhage leading to an improvement in department's management of the condition).
- Students interaction with you (e.g. they appear interested).
- You are invited back to do more teaching.

# TELL ME ABOUT YOUR RESEARCH EXPERIENCE

- If you have been involved in research, explain why you did it and your findings.
- If you have not been involved in research, explain any exposure you may have had to research skills and if you want to do research in the future.
    - Example 1: I have not performed any research projects, however, as a doctor I think it is extremely important to be able to critically appraise research so that an evidence-based approach can be used to provide the best care for patients. To enhance this skill, I have therefore been attending a journal club regularly.
    - Example 2: An example of where I have used evidence based medicine is...
- Be able to discuss a recent research paper (you may be asked about a research paper that has impacted your management or a recent paper that you have read).

# SHOULD EVERYONE DO RESEARCH?

- It does not matter which side you favor, as long as you present well-balanced arguments for both sides and explain the pros and cons.

- NO?
  - Taking time out to do research means time out from clinical duties and if research lasts for a long time, there is a danger of losing skills.
  - Limited funding and resources for research – therefore better for more enthusiastic people to do research so as to gain maximum contribution and advancement to the field.
  - However, important to be able to understand how research is conducted and critically appraise findings.

- YES?
  - Enables doctors to better understand and appraise research papers and therefore practice evidence based medicine.
  - Contribute to medical advancement.

# AUDIT VERSUS RESEARCH

**AUDIT:**
Comparing clinical practice against set standards.

**RESEARCH**:
Creating new knowledge (which may be used to develop standards).

- Therefore research establishes what the best practice should be, and audit assesses whether we are applying this best practice to our clinical activities.

| | |
|---|---|
| **Why is audit important?** | • One of the seven pillars of clinical governance<br>• Ensures quality of care maintained at an agreed standard.<br>• Encourages better use of resources and improved efficiency. |
| **Why is research important?** | • Drives medical advancement by developing a pool of knowledge which can be translated into better patient care. |

# TELL ME ABOUT AN AUDIT THAT YOU HAVE DONE

- Explain your audit using the audit cycle:
  - Identify an issue.
  - Identify the standard.
  - Collect data on current practice.
  - Compare current practice to standards.
  - Implement change.
  - Re-audit.
  - Present the audit.

## EXAMPLE:

I realised that antibiotic prescribing was not being done as well as it should be. I therefore looked up the Trust standards for antibiotic prescribing, and created a proforma with which I collected data from one hundred patients. This showed a suboptimal adherence to trust guidelines and poor documentation of the duration and reasoning for antibiotics. I presented the results at a departmental meeting and produced posters to raise awareness. A re-audit showed significant improvement, completing the audit loop.

# LEADERSHIP VERSUS MANAGEMENT

**LEADER**
Sets direction/vision and directs others towards that goal.

**MANAGER**
Manages the resources to achieve it.

## EXAMPLE OF LEADERSHIP AND MANAGEMENT

As a medical student, I realised how stressful final year OSCEs (Objective structured clinical examinations) can be and how important it is to identify areas of improvement early on. As a foundation year doctor, I therefore decided to organise a mock OSCE for final year medical students. This involved writing 21 scenarios and mark schemes, organising room bookings, finding patients willing to be examined and the hardest part - encouraging doctors to take an evening out of their free time to examine students. The mock-OSCE ran very well and received excellent feedback. I was awarded a leadership award for my contribution.

# TELL ME ABOUT A WEAKNESS OF YOURS

- The dreaded question!!
- Use a weakness that has a positive spin and always end on a positive note.

## EXAMPLE 1

I am a very enthusiastic and motivated person. This does however sometimes mean that I end up taking on too many projects at one time, which can become quite stressful and difficult to manage. E.g. Last year whilst working I was also (list other projects/activities). After reflecting on this weakness, I now make sure that I fully appreciate what other projects I have on, before undertaking new projects and if in doubt, speak to my educational supervisor.

## EXAMPLE 2

I am a very caring and empathetic person. However, due to this nature, I can sometimes become too emotionally attached to patients. For example, during my last rotation, a patient who had been under our care for six weeks passed away. I found this very upsetting/distressing. When this happened, I reflected and spoke to my seniors for advice. I learnt the importance of remaining empathetic but at the same time keeping an appropriate emotional distance and I hope to develop this skill further during my training.

# TELL US ABOUT A MISTAKE YOU HAVE MADE

- Ensure you discuss the following:
  - Patient safety is your priority so rectify your mistake.
  - Inform senior.
  - Be honest with patient and apologise.
  - Reflect.
  - Take steps to prevent recurrence.
    - Example 1) Discuss at teaching/departmental meetings.
    - Example 2) Make a proforma to ensure this aspect is not missed again.
  - Submit a incident report if appropriate to ensure that the hospital or department as a whole can learn from the mistake.

# WHAT ARE YOUR SKILLS IN TEAMWORK/LEADERSHIP/ COMMUNICATION/EMPATHY?

- Expect at least one question in this area
- Have a specific example that highlights you
- What have you learned and how will you carry this forward to your ST1 job?
- E.g. Teamwork
    - ***Set the scene:*** As an FY1/2 on my acute medicine job, I was part of the weekend on call ward cover team. This included 1 registrar, 2 SHOs and 1 FY1 covering all the wards, tasked with reviewing about 150 patients in 12 hour shift.
    - ***What skills did you learn:*** We had morning huddle, allocate patients or wards to each person, aware of everyone's role and limitations e.g. FY1 would not see ITU step downs. We would meet every 3-4 hours to talk about what jobs were completed, if we needed support with our workload. Taught me importance of good communication, knowing your role, being able to delegate, carrying out your role in a team efficiently.
    - ***How will it help you in ST1:*** Important skills on labour ward: working with MDT (consultants, registrars, anaesthetists, paediatricians, midwives, support staff).

# HOW DO YOU HANDLE STRESS?

- How do you handle stress inside your job?
  - Give a specific example of a stressful situation - e.g. responding to an emergency, managing a busy on call, taking care of an unwell patient
  - What strategies did you use to cope – e.g. follow a structured approach, ask for help from a senior, delegate, prioritise your tasks
  - What happened afterwards – reflect on the situation, comment on positive feedback from a consultant/registrar or patient, what was the learning point from the situation
- What do you do to de-stress outside your job?
  - Good time to talk about your extracurriculars/hobbies
  - Important to maintain a good work life balance' – high attrition rates in O&G
- Show them you have a realistic understanding of demanding nature of this job

# MBRRACE REPORT

- MBRRACE: Mothers and Babies - Reducing Risk through Audits and Confidential Enquiries across the UK
- MBRRACE is a collaboration appointed by the Healthcare Quality Improvement Partnership, which investigates maternal deaths, stillbirths, and infant deaths.
- The MBRRACE-UK Saving Lives Report is a MUST READ document
- Try and bring points from the MBRRACE report into your answers.

## Summary of the MBRRACE-UK Saving Lives 2019 Report:

- The MBRRACE Confidential Enquiry into Maternal Deaths report assesses maternal mortality over a three year period. The latest report was published in December 2019, which looks at maternal mortality from 2015-2017.
- Maternal death rate is defined as the death of a woman while pregnant or within 6 weeks of delivery/termination of pregnancy (excluding accidental or incidental causes)
- There has been a statistically non-significant decrease in the overall maternal death rate in the UK between 2012-14 and 2015-17 (maternal death rate of 9.16 versus 9.78 per 100,000 maternities).
- Indirect deaths are defined as deaths resulting from pre-existing disease, or disease that developed during pregnancy and which were not the result of direct obstetric causes, but which were aggravated by the physiological effects of pregnancy.
- Direct causes are deaths occurring from obstetric complications of pregnancy (e.g. haemorrhage).
- During this triennium, causes of death in order of incidence were:
    1. Cardiac causes (indirect)
    2. Thrombosis and thromboembolism (direct)
    3. Neurological (indirect)
    4. Other indirect (indirect)
    5. Sepsis (direct/indirect depending on source of sepsis)
    6. Psychiatric (suicide is a direct cause, drugs/alcohol is an indirect cause)

## MBRRACE-UK Saving Lives 2017 Report (Continued):

- Key area of improvement highlighted by the report include:
  - Improving care of women with cardiovascular disease
  - Improving care of women with breast cancer in pregnancy
  - Improving care of women with pre-eclampsia and hypertensive disorders of pregnancy
  - Improving care of women with early pregnancy disorders
  - Lessons from accidental deaths in pregnancy and the postpartum period
  - Messages for critical care

**NOTES**

- Deaths due to indirect causes still remain the major proportion (58%) of maternal deaths in the UK.
- The direct maternal death rate has decreased by 44% since 2003-05 with a 26% decrease in the rate of indirect maternal deaths
- The reducing maternal mortality rate is predominantly due to a decrease in maternal deaths from haemorrhage and amniotic fluid embolism.
- There has been a statistically non-significant increase in mortality rate from neurological causes (stroke/epilepsy), now making it the the third commonest cause of death overall.
- Maternal suicide is the second largest cause of direct maternal deaths occurring during or within 6 weeks of the end of pregnancy and remains the leading cause of direct deaths occurring within a year after the end of pregnancy.
- There remains a five-fold difference in maternal mortality rates amongst women from Black ethnic backgrounds and an almost two-fold difference amongst women from Asian ethnic backgrounds focus on actions to address these disparities. compared to white women, emphasising the need for a continued focus on action to address these disparities.

## MBRRACE-UK Perinatal Mortality Report

MBRRACE-UK also investigates perinatal mortality and publishes yearly reports on this subject. The last report was published in October 2019, which assessed perinatal mortality between January to December 2017.

**Key points:**

- The extended perinatal mortality rate (from 24 weeks of pregnancy until 4 weeks after birth) in UK was 5.40 deaths per 1,000 births. This has reduced from 6.04 deaths per 1,000 total births in 2013.
- The stillbirth rate (a baby delivered at or after 24+0 weeks gestational age showing no signs of life) for the UK has reduced from 4.20 to 3.74 per 1,000 births from 2013 to 2017.
- The largest fall in stillbirth and neonatal death rates is seen in term babies (37+0 to 41+6 weeks gestational age), accounting for half of the reduction seen in these rates.
- Mortality rates remain higher for Black/Black British/Asian or Asian British babies.
- There is an increasing national focus on reducing perinatal mortality with a number of national initiatives.
- These national initiatives include:
    - Each Baby Counts (The Royal College of Obstetricians and Gynaecologists - RCOG)
    - Saving Babies' Lives Care Bundle (NHS England)
    - 1000 Lives Improvement, National Stillbirth Working Group (NHS Wales)
    - Maternity and Children's Quality Improvement Collaborative (NHS Scotland)
    - The Northern Ireland Maternal and Infant Loss (NIMI) steering group.

# EACH BABY COUNTS INITIATIVE

Each Baby Counts is a UK-wide quality improvement programme led by the Royal College of Obstetricians and Gynaecologists (RCOG). Its aim is to reduce the incidence of intrapartum stillbirth, early neonatal death and severe brain injury as a result of events in labour by 50% between 2015 and 2020.

All NHS trusts in the UK report eligible babies to the Each Baby Counts Initiative. Eligible babies include all term babies (at least 37+0 completed weeks of gestation) born following labour who have one of the following outcomes: Intrapartum stillbirth, early neonatal death or severe brain injury. Anonymised reports from local review are then sent to two independent Each Baby Counts reviewers - a midwife and an obstetrician. The reviewers do not have access to the case notes or statements from the staff involved; therefore the process is reliant upon the quality of the local reviews. Learning from these cases are collaborated into Each Baby Counts reports where recommendations are made.

The key benefit of the Each Baby Counts Initiative is that the scenarios reviewed are rare in individual maternity units, and therefore it is difficult to see clear patterns or identify how best to avoid them. The Each Baby Counts programme brings together the results of local investigations to help understand the bigger picture, share the lessons learned and prevent babies from dying or sustaining brain injuries in the future.

## KEY RECOMMENDATIONS:

### Workload

The labour ward coordinator must remain supernumerary at all times and should not be caring for women during the antenatal, intrapartum or postnatal period.

### Escalating High Activity

There must be a clear escalation policy in place and a culture that empowers staff to escalate when the workload is becoming difficult to manage. All members of staff, irrespective of their role or grade, should feel empowered to inform senior midwives, managers and consultants when concerns arise both within their own specialty but also on behalf of another specialty. The consultant obstetrician should always be informed when labour ward activity is high.

### Cross-Site Communication

Women receiving care from multiple units must have an individualised management plan for antenatal, labour and postnatal care that outlines the roles and responsibilities of each site to avoid any confusion. All sites should be able to readily access a woman's notes whether they be hand-held or electronic.

### Local Guidelines

There must be a clear policy to ensure that local guidelines are updated in line with national guidance. Appropriate resources and staff time must be allocated to facilitate this. Where units decide to deviate from national guidance, this should be clearly documented and units should undertake regular review of local deviations from national guidance. All guidelines should be reviewed in light of incidents to ensure that they improve care as intended.

## Migration of Boundaries

Teams should protect against migration of boundaries by ensuring that real practice reflects practice as described in guidelines. Audit identifies where migrations from safe practice are occurring, but it is only through a process of quality improvement or changing unworkable guidelines that these migrations can be corrected.

## Anaesthetic Care

A decision about the purpose of transfer to theatre and urgency of any birth should be made together with the anaesthetist before transfer to theatre. The degree of urgency should be reviewed on entering theatre before the WHO check, and the obstetrician should confirm the degree of urgency directly to the anaesthetist.

# THE NHS LONG TERM PLAN

In 2018, the government announced £20.5bn of additional funding for the NHS in England by 2023/24. The NHS Long Term Plan launched in January 2019 sets out priorities for how this money will be spent over the next ten years.

**The features relevant to Obstetrics and Gynaecology, include:**

- Reducing stillbirths and mother and child deaths during birth by 50%
- Ensuring most women can benefit from continuity of care through and beyond their pregnancy, targeted towards those who will benefit most
- Providing extra support for expectant mothers at risk of premature birth
- Expanding support for perinatal mental health conditions

# BETTER FOR WOMEN REPORT

The Royal College of Obstetricians and Gynaecologists (RCOG) is calling for better joined up services, as part of its "Better for Women" report, published in November 2019.

### THE KEY POINTS RECOMMENDATIONS IN THE REPORT ARE:

**Access to reliable information on women's health**

E.g. The NHS website should become the world's best source of information for girls, women and clinicians

**Easy access to contraception, abortion and fertility services**

E.g. Post-pregnancy contraception should be a key part of the maternity pathway

E.g. End post-code lotteries in IVF treatment and offer all eligible women three full cycles of IVF

**Learning from indicators in the reproductive years to influence future health**

E.g. Improve identification of women at risk from mental and physical health issues with the six week postnatal check

**End violence against girls and women**

E.g. End violence against girls and women via an improved collaborative approach, better IT systems and mandatory training with the NHS as an exemplar

**Prevention of mortality from gynaecological cancers across the life course**

E.g. Increase uptake in cervical screening amongst disadvantaged and marginalised women including implementation of HPV primary home-test screening.

**Keeping women in the workforce**

E.g. Women's health issues should be embedded in workplace policies

# NHS LITIGATION AUTHORITY (NHSLA)

A special health authority which handles negligence claims made against NHS bodies in England, and has an active risk management programme to help raise standards of care in the NHS and reduce the number of incidents leading to claims. It produces an annual report detailing the number of clinical negligence claims that year according to medical specialty.

The 2015/16 report shows that 10% of all claims made during that 12 month period related to obstetrics, making it the third most litigious area of medicine. Gynaecology was the fifth most common area, making up 6% of clinical negligence claims.

In terms of value, however, obstetrics was clearly the most expensive. The total value of claims received during 2015/16 was £2,896,367,802, and 42% of this figure could be attributed to obstetric claims. Gynaecology was just 3% of the figure.

# BURNOUT IN OBSTETRICS AND GYNAECOLOGY

A nationwide study released in November 2019 found that 36% of obstetricians and gynaecologists met the criteria for burnout and were six times more likely to experience suicidal thoughts, four times more likely to report depression, and three times more likely to report anxiety, irritability and anger. They also suffered from sleep and relationship problems.

Obstetricians and gynaecologists with burnout were four times more likely to practice 'defensively' – meaning a doctor may avoid difficult cases or procedures, over prescribe medications, or carry out more investigations or treatments than necessary, for fear of making a mistake or missing a diagnosis.

In response to this, the RCOG have established a 'Supporting our Doctors' task group, which includes a 'peer to peer' support service and a network of workforce champions to provide pastoral and practical support to doctors and employers.

# STRUCTURED INTERVIEW - MARK SCHEME

| | |
|---|---|
| Understanding and commitment to the specialty:<br>• Why do you want to pursue a career in Obstetrics and Gynaecology?<br>• What are your training priorities for the first 12 months?<br>• What challenges do trainees in Obstetrics and Gynaecology face and how would you overcome these?<br>• How have you shown commitment to the specialty?<br>• How is Obstetrics and Gynaecology changing as a specialty? | /5 |
| Experience outside obstetrics and gynaecology, team-working and leadership:<br>• What extra-curricular activities do you do and how will they help you in this specialty?<br>• What is your biggest achievement and how does this apply to a career in Obstetrics and Gynaecology?<br>• Give me an example of where you have worked well in a team<br>• Give me an example of where you have shown leadership skills<br>• What is your biggest weakness?<br>• Tell me about a mistake you have made | /5 |
| Quality improvement measures:<br>• Tell me about an audit or quality improvement project you have done? Did you close the loop/re-audit?<br>• What is the difference between audit and research? | /5 |
| Teaching and research experience:<br>• Have you done any research?<br>• Do you think everyone should do research?<br>• Tell me about you teaching experience?<br>• How do you know that you are a good teacher? | /5 |
| Total | /20 |

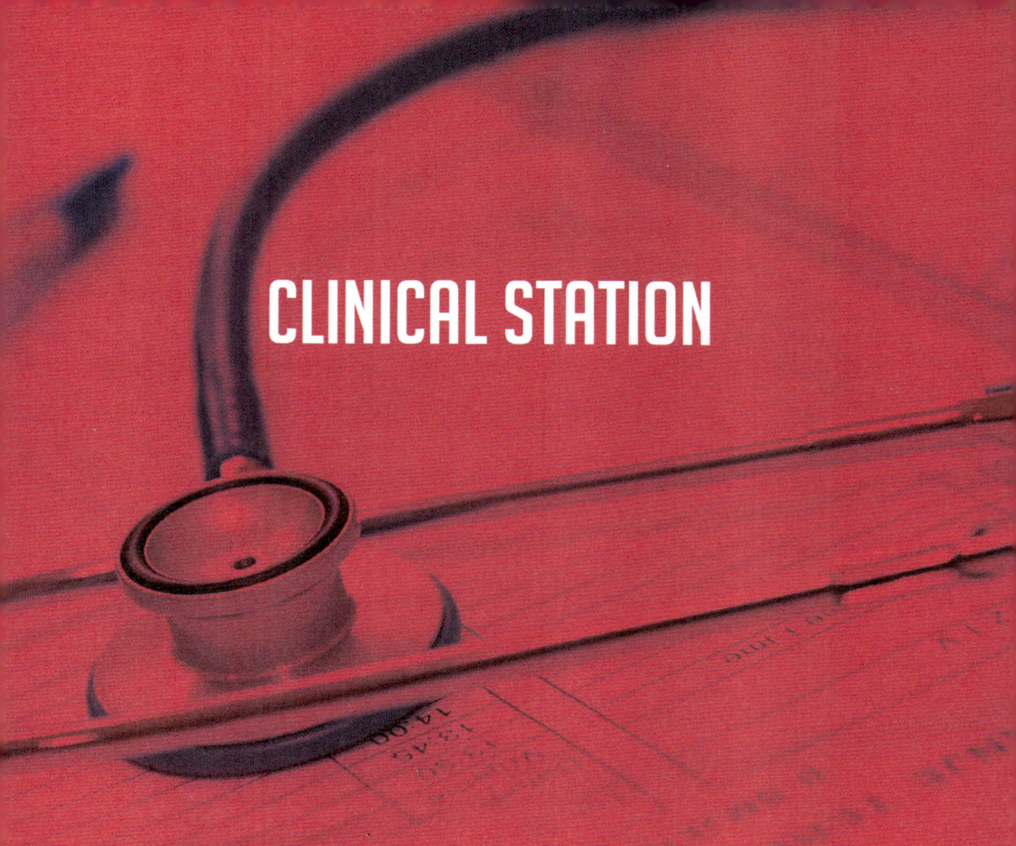

# CLINICAL STATION

OBSTETRICS AND GYNAECOLOGY ST1
INTERVIEW BOOK

obsandgynae.net

# CLINICAL SKILLS PRESENTATION

- You are given four to five clinical scenarios and are tasked with prioritising and managing these patients. In the past few years the scenarios have moved away from obstetrics/gynaecology towards general medical/surgical situations.
- Structure of the station - you will be given:
  - The list of patients (4-5) that you have to deal with
  - Their observations (HR, BP, RR, O2 saturations, temperature
  - A team that can help you (Gynaecology registrar, Orthopaedic Registrar, FY1)
  - The examiners will not give you any further information or engage with your discussion. They will only listen, clarify and mark you.

It can be intimidating to speak for 15 minutes - remember: the examiners will not react to what you say.

## IMPORTANT TIPS

1. If anyone is acutely unwell, ALWAYS seek senior help (O&G registrar/ consultant, A and E consultant if in A and E, anaesthetic consultant, Medical or surgical registrars)
2. Escalate but only if it is appropriate use of staffing
3. Think about who else can help you e.g. –
   - If cannula is needed – do you have an FY1/site nurse practitioner
   - If someone is pregnant but having an asthma attack in A and E – A and E team can review
   - If someone most likely has appendicitis, surgical team to review
   - If a relative is asking about a patient's progress the sister in charge can help
   - If an urgent discharge summary needs doing- FY1 can help
   - If you're busy reviewing a sick patient, you can ask nurse to start management plan until you get there e.g. give PRN analgesia already on the drug chart to someone with post-op pain

# YOUR APPROACH

It is very important to be able to answer/ask yourself the following questions about each scenario:

- Which patient is my priority?
- How do I assess the patient?
- What investigations do I order and why?
- How am I going to stabilise the patient?
- What do I think the differential diagnosis is?
- What am I going to do next?

# COMMON THEMES

- Upper gastrointestinal bleed
- Post-op pain
- Transfusion reaction
- Acute limb ischaemia
- Chest pain
- Infection/sepsis
- Confused patient
- Ruptured appendix

# EXAMPLE SCENARIO

You have received the following bleeps within a 5 minute period. Please read through the scenarios below and then discuss with the examiner about how you will prioritise the scenarios below.

- Patient 1: 45-year-old male on surgical ward with haematemesis. Observations: BP90/40, HR120bpm, 96% RA, RR24, T36.1
- Patient 2: 23-year-old female on orthopaedic ward having blood transfusion post-op, having a fever. Observations: BP120/80, HR90bpm, 100% RA, RR18, T38.0
- Patient 3: 88-year-old lady with pain after hip fracture fixation. Observations: BP 130/80, HR 80bpm, 98% RA, RR17, T37.2
- Son of Patient 3 calls you requesting an update on his mother.

The following people are available to assist you: General Surgical Registrar, Orthopaedic Registrar, Gynaecology Registrar, FY1.

## UPPER GI BLEED (PATIENT 1)

- Number 1 priority
- I would ask the nurse how much EBL has been
- Start your ABCDE assessment (talk through this) and resuscitate the patient

A - I would speak to the patient, ensure their airway was patent

B - they are tachypneic which can indicate significant blood loss.

- I would listen to their chest, assess air entry (for signs of aspiration from vomiting).
- Administer 15 L of oxygen via a non-rebreathe mask.

C - they are tachycardic and hypotensive which is concerning.
I would check if they appeared pale and had cold peripheries.

- Insert 2 large bore cannula
- Take blood samples: FBC, U&E, LFTs, Clotting, VBG (to obtain quick Hb)
- Group & Save and Crossmatch - at least 2-4 units
- Give IV fluids stat
- As they are haemodynamically unstable with ongoing bleeding, appropriate to consider "major haemorrhage protocol" and give O- blood
- Monitor urine output, commence fluid balance chart
- CXR - pneumoperitoneum

D - check their consciousness level using GCS/AVPU

E - to complete your assessment:

- Abdomen - check for guarding, signs of peritonism, hepatomegaly

- Differentials: Peptic ulcer perforation, Mallory-Weiss Tear, Variceal bleeding, Malignancy
- What next:
  - Escalate to your seniors - in this case, General Surgical Registrar
  - Contact Anaesthetist as patient may need to go to theatre for endoscopy

## TRANSFUSION REACTION (PATIENT 2)

- Number 2 priority as patient haemodynamically stable
- As you are with Patient 1, ask nurse to stop the transfusion immediately. If any concerning features e.g. hypoxia/hypotension, nurse can put out 2222 call
- Ensure transfusion is stopped, don't use transfusion IV line and do not flush
- When you arrive, start your ABCDE assessment to exclude severe reactions
  - A - check airway is patent (anaphylaxis)
  - B - assess for dyspnoea or stridor (anaphylaxis), hypoxia (TRALI)
  - C - assess for hypotension/shock/collapse/reduced urine output (bacterial contamination, acute haemolytic reaction) - if you suspect haemolysis send FBC/LDH/Bilirubin/Clotting. Cultures on patient and product if you think bacterial contamination. G&S.
- Differentials: Febrile non-haemolytic transfusion reaction, Bacterial contamination, Acute haemolytic transfusion reaction, Anaphylaxis, TRALI
- Febrile non-haemolytic reaction:
  - Mild: If temperature ≥ 38.0°C or rise of 1-2°C, itching/rash only you can continue the transfusion. Treat symptoms i.e. chlorphenamine. Monitor closely for any deterioration.
  - Moderate: If temperature ≥ 39.0°C or rise of >2°C, think bacterial contamination. IV antibiotics if sepsis.
- You can mention if anaphylaxis suspected: 2222, Adrenaline 0.5mg IM, Hydrocortisone 200mg IV, Chlorphenamine 10mg IV, IV fluids stat.

# POST-OP PAIN (PATIENT 3)

- Number 3 priority
- Haemodynamically stable, not febrile
- You can send your FY1 to review the patient
- Give them advise on what to look for:
  - A-E assessment
  - Exclude common post-op complications: DVT, infection, bleeding
  - Ensure their analgesia is appropriate, analgesia ladder
- Afterwards, you should get handover from FY1

# CONFIDENTIALITY (PATIENT 4)

- Number 4 priority
- You don't have to speak to the son yourself - remember to delegate! Can be nurse in charge, FY1 etc.
- Ensure that you have the patient's permission first, and what they would like disclosed
- "Trust is an essential part of the doctor-patient relationship and confidentiality is central to this."
- "Doctors are under both ethical and legal duties to protect patients' personal information."
- When can you disclose patient's information?
  - With patient's consent
  - If patient lacks capacity to consent
  - Permitted by law
  - Under legal process
  - In the public interest

# ACUTE CONFUSION

78 Year old patient confused day 2 following Neck Of Femur fracture. Obs BP 100/50, HR 120, Temp 38.9, stats 94%, RR 20. O/E patient is flushed, clammy and disorientated. How would you manage?

- Explain why you are concerned: tachycardic, hypotensive, febrile, tachypneic.
- ABCDE assessment. Discuss your examination systematically for each component
  1. Respiratory - listen to the chest
  2. Cardiovascular - heart sounds, capillary refills
  3. Abdominal examination - any distention, mention guarding and rebound tenderness. Check for bowel sounds, ask about passing flatus.
  4. Examine any operation site
  5. Examine the calves bilaterally – check if soft, tender, oedaematous, erythematous
  6. Examine for any rashes
  7. Examine ears, nose, throat
  8. Muscular skeletal examinations, assessing power/tone/sensation, co-ordination
  9. Genitourinary exam
- Investigations:
  - FBC, CRP, U&Es, lactate
  - Urine dipstick and mid stream urine
  - ECG as tachycardia
  - Chest x-ray
  - Arterial blood gas
  - Swabs from operative site/other relevant cultures such as sputum, high vaginal swab
  - Imaging including imaging from operative site

- Management:
  - Put the patient on high flow oxygen
  - Gain intravenous access
  - Give intravenous fluids
  - Commence intravenous antibiotics and paracetamol
  - Catheterise, send mid stream urine and commence an input and output chart

## TALK THROUGH IT

"I'll introduce myself to the patient and confirm his details. This will allow me to know he is alert and his airway is patent."

"I will begin to do a complete physical examination"

"As he is tachycardic, hypotensive and febrile, I will insert two large bore cannulas (Grey), take blood cultures and bloods for FBC, U&Es, CRP, I will prescribe and give 1L IV fluid STAT and after confirming allergy status, I will start IV antibiotics per local guidelines "

"I will ask or a blood glucose to rule out hypoglycaemia"

"I will ask for the patient to be catheterized, check a urine dipstick and send off mid stream urine"

"I will send of a sputum culture if the patient has a productive cough"

"I will ask for an ECG as the patient is tachycardic and, I will do an ABG and Chest X-ray as tachypneic"

**Differential diagnosis of acute confusion include:**

- Sepsis
- Urinary Retention
- Pulmonary embolism
- TIA
- Hypoglycaemia
- Drug misuse
- Alcohol withdrawal

# POST-OP INFECTION

A 32 year old lady attends A and E five days following caesarean section feeling generally unwell. T 38.5, BP 110/86, P 110, RR 16, O2 saturations 100% on air

- Observations suggest she is SEPTIC therefore inform A and E consultant/anaesthetist and move her into resus.
- Carry out septic six
  - Intravenous access and fluids
  - Urinary catheter and measure urine output
  - FBC, U and E, CRP and lactate, blood cultures
  - Other cultures including MSU, swabs from surgical site, high vaginal swab, throat swab
  - Intravenous antibiotics
  - Oxygen
- Inform registrar/consultant

# FULL ASSESSMENT:

- Listen to chest, examine breasts, palpate abdomen (wound site, is uterus well contracted), speculum examination and swabs), and examine legs (PE can cause raised temperature)
- Empirical antibiotics: cefuroxime and metronidazole broad spectrum and safe in breastfeeding but check trust guidelines/liaise with microbiologist for advice
- Potential sources of infection: Endometritis, retained products of pregnancy, urinary tract infection, chest sepsis, mastitis.

# POST-OP INFECTION (2)

58 year old lady, day 1 post anterior/posterior repair and TVT for a uterine prolapse. The nurses on Gynaecology ward bleep you, because the patient doesn't look well and complaining of abdominal pain. Obs BP 100/50, R 120, Temp 38.9, stats 94%, RR 20. O/E patient is flushed, clammy. How would you manage?

- ABCDE
- Perform a systemic examination, including VE/speculum
- Conduct the SEPTIC SIX.
- Resuscitate the patient and commence antibiotics.
- Mention vaginal pack - that you will look for any retained packs that could be source of infection (DDX: Post op sepsis secondary to vaginal pack)
- Remove the source of infection:
    - 15mins obs
    - Inform seniors
    - If the patient spikes again d/w microbiologist

# SEPSIS 6

- A pathway which should be delivered within one hour of the diagnosis of sepsis.

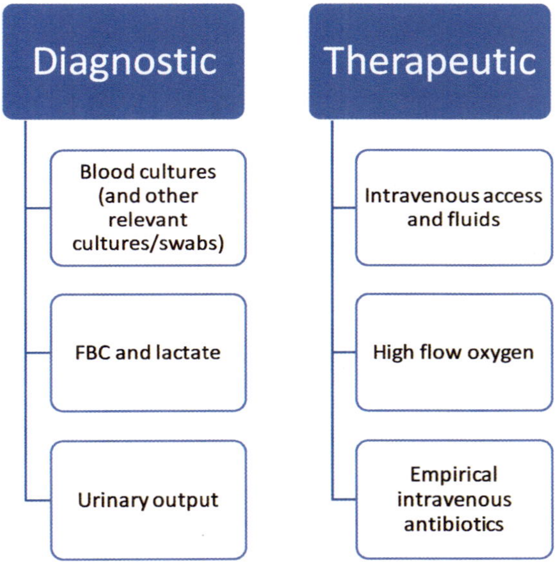


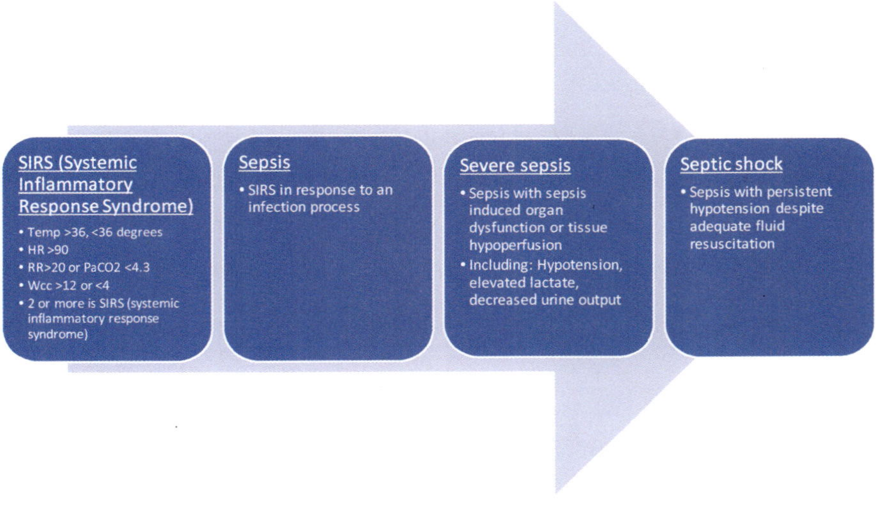

# POST-OPERATIVE BLEED

45 year old, day 0 post total laparoscopic hysterectomy for menorrhagia with reduced urine output. P 110, BP 100/65, afebrile, 100% on air, RR 18. How would you manage?

- In your ABCDE assessment you should also look for:
  - Assess abdomen for peritonism, scar site tenderness, PV bleeding?
  - Reduced urine out
  - Pre-op Hb, any post-op Hb
  - EBL
  - Review op notes: any surgical complications? any drains in situ?
  - If any drains left, what is the output
- Tell nurse you are coming immediately, but in the meantime if patient has IV access, to put up a bag of Hartmann's
- Urgently call registrar/consultant and anaesthetist as likely needs to go to theatre.
- Remember to delegate: ask nurse to call theatre, porters and blood bank and cross match four units. If delay in receiving blood (e.g. not already group and saved) ask for O negative
- Check what analgesia they are on , and give further analgesia if require

# SIMILAR SCENARIOS:

- Post-op pain - If observations are stable, no signs of bleeding, good urine output, minimal drain output and not on analgesia can ask FY1 to assess and prescribe analgesia (and to inform you if further concerns)
- Reduced urine output – If observations are stable, no signs of bleeding, minimal drain output, can ask nurse to flush catheter to ascertain if genuine poor urine output or blocked catheter and urinary retention causing pain.

# POST-OPERATIVE THROMBOSIS

65 year old patient on the orthopedic ward following ankle operation day 3, complaining of right leg pain and leg swelling. HR 88, BP 100/60, afebrile, RR 25, Sats 95%. How would you manage?

- ABCDE assessment
- Check for tenderness/erythematous swollen calf
- Ensure intravenous access
- Send bloods incl FBC, U and E, CRP, ABG
- Mention patient's risk factors - post op, over weight, smoker, not on thromboprophylaxis!
- Treat as thromboembolic disease
- Weigh patient, commence treatment dose LMWH as per guidelines
- Inform your senior
- Urgent USS doppler

# CONFIDENTIALITY

**The haematology consultant asks about his mother's CT results which shows metastasis. How would you manage?**

- Apologize to the son and express you can not breach patient confidentiality.
- The son can directly speak to his mother regarding the results of her investigations.
- With patient's consent, he can attend the morning ward round to learn about his mother's progress.
- If you are not able to speak to the son directly, delegate the above task to the ward sister.

# MENTAL HEALTH AND PREGNANCY

24 year old female presenting to A&E with left sided severe abdominal pain and PV bleeding. Her observations are: HR 120 bpm, BP 90/50, RR 18, 98% on RA, T36.3. Urine - dipstick negative, BHCG positive.

- Patient is high priority, haemodynamically unstable - therefore, you will attend urgently to review her.
- A-E assessment and resuscitate patient, talk through each stage of the A-E assessment and focus closely on:
    - 2 large bore cannulas
    - Bloods to be sent off - FBC, U&E, CRP, Clotting, 2 Group and Saves and VBG
    - Cross match 4 units
    - Fluid resuscitation - 1L Hartmann's stat
    - Give O negative blood if continues to be haemodynamically unstable
- Examine looking for signs of peritonism, and speculum examination for severity of bleeding
- Impression: Likely ruptured ectopic pregnancy, needs urgent senior review +/- theatre
- Discuss with registrar/consultant whether patient is suitable for ultrasound if stable (to confirm ectopic and look for any haemoperitoneum), or whether she needs to go to theatre directly
- If unstable and going to theatre, inform: emergency theatre staff, anaesthetist, porters, blood bank, and keep patient nil by mouth
- Management: after immediate resuscitation, definitive management will include urgent surgery - either salpingectomy/salpingotomy, laparoscopically or open.

# PELVIC INFLAMMATORY DISEASE

30 year old female presents to A&E with left iliac fossa pain and offensive discharge. Her observations are: HR 110bpm, BP 90/40, RR 25, 98% on RA, T39.5. Urine dip and HCG - negative.

- High priority patient as there are signs she is septic - you will need to review her urgently
- A-E assessment and resuscitate patient. Talk through each stage of the assessment with the examiner, and focus closely on:
  - Sepsis Six - GIVE: IV fluids, Broad spectrum antibiotics, High flow oxygen. TAKE: Blood culture, lactate, urine output
  - Additionally, send off: FBC, CRP, U&E, LFT
  - Cultures: urine, high vaginal and endocervical swab
  - Examine: abdomen - renal angle tenderness, guarding; vaginal examination - cervical excitation, adnexal tenderness
- Impression: Differentials include pyelonephritis (unlikely with negative urine dip), or pelvic inflammatory disease
- History taking should include - gynaecological history, exploring risk factors such as sexual history, previous sexually transmitted infections, pelvic surgery, intrauterine coils
- Management: after Sepsis Six, arrange ultrasound scan looking for tubo-ovarian abscess and free fluid. Surgically, may need drainage if large abscess or continues to be unwell with no improvement on IV Antibiotics.

# MISCARRIAGE

25 year old female presents to Early Pregnancy Unit with heavy vaginal bleeding. Her observations are: HR 80bpm, BP 110/80, RR 18, 98% on RA, T37.3. She is 8/40 with confirmed intrauterine pregnancy on ultrasound scan last week.

- Haemodynamically stable
- A-E assessment, focusing closely on:
  - Abdomen - signs of guarding or peritonism
  - Speculum - assesses for severity of bleeding, clots, products of pregnancy
  - Types of miscarriages:
    1. Threatened - bleeding, closed cervix, USS – Intra-uterine pregnancy and fetal heart seen
    2. Complete - bleeding stops, closed cervix, USS - empty uterus
    3. Incomplete - bleeding, open cervix, USS - tissue or gestational sac
    4. Missed - bleeding, closed cervix, USS – pregnancy with no fetal heart seen
- Management of miscarriage:
  - Initial resuscitation, including blood products and IV fluids if haemodynamically unstable. Ultrasound scan looking for fetal heart and products of conception. Following this, can offer patient options of expectant, medical or surgical management of miscarriage.
  - Expectant: possible if no heavy bleeding. May take several weeks. Can offer repeat scan to confirm complete miscarriage
  - Medical: Oral or vaginal misoprostol, mifepristone. Risk of heavy bleeding and requiring ERPC.
  - Surgical: ERPC especially if heavy bleeding. If haemodynamically unstable will need to go to theatre urgently. Risks of infection, perforation, retained products.

# CLINICAL STATION 1

You are the FY2 on call and have received the following bleeps within a 5 minute period. Please read through the scenarios below and then discuss with the examiner about how you will prioritise the scenarios below. The Medical Registrar, Orthopaedic Registrar, Gynaecology Registrar and FY1 can be contacted

A. 65-year-old Mr A, on the orthopedic ward four days following a hip operation, complaining of lower leg pain and swelling. Observations: Heart rate 110, temperature 36.7, respiratory rate 16, oxygen Saturation 96%, blood pressure 110/72.

B. 98-year-old Mrs B, on the medical ward, admitted with acute confusion. Observations: Heart rate 120, blood pressure 90/60, respiratory rate 22, afebrile.

C. 45-year-old, Mrs C, day 0 post total laparoscopic hysterectomy for menorrhagia with reduced urine output. Observations: Heart rate 120, blood pressure 72/48, temperature 36, respiratory rate 22, oxygen saturations 100 percent on air.

D. A local newspaper reporter calls and asks about a famous patient on the ward.

E. 35-year-old Mrs E, post laparoscopic myomectomy with abdominal pain, with PCA needs a new cannula. Observations: Stable, good urine output, 20ml in drain, blood loss in theatre minimal.

# CLINICAL STATION 1 - MARK SCHEME

| | |
|---|---|
| Rapid assessment and prioritisation (CABED) | /5 |
| Appropriate management of Mr A:<br>• Investigations: Leg Doppler USS<br>• Impression: Likely Deep Vein Thrombosis, post operation.<br>• Management: If patient was on prophylactic thrombolytic drugs, if yes stop and commence treatment dose thrombolytics i.e. Heparin or Fragmin. If not on thromboprophylaxis, do a Datix from, as patients' VTE assessment not done accurately. | /5 |
| Appropriate management of Mrs B:<br>• Investigations: Urine dip, send MSU/CXR, bloods; FBC, U&E, CRP<br>• Impression: Infection<br>• Management: Full assessment - cardiorespiratory, CNS, GI, ENT, Urogenital. Confirm allergy status, and commence antibiotics based on local protocol. IV access and IV fluids. If patient spikes temperature, to do full septic screen and liaise with microbiologist/inform seniors.<br>• Other causes of confusion in elderly. Sepsis, Urinary Retention, Hypoxia (?PE), TIA, Hypoglycaemia, Drug misuse, Alcohol withdrawal. | /5 |
| Appropriate management of Mrs C:<br>• Identifies that Mrs C should be prioritised and seen first. Establishes that they need senior review.<br>• Impression: UNSTABLE, needs to see FIRST. Post-operative bleed.<br>• Management – Inform seniors/operating team and anaesthetist. Ensure two large bore cannulae, intravenous fluids, oxygen, bloods including full blood count, group and save and venous blood gas for immediate haemoglobin. Cross match 4 units.<br>• Blood tests/gas to look for signs of anaemia secondary to haemorrhage, raised lactate and metabolic acidosis secondary to heamorrhagic shock/sepsis.<br>• If stabilises, consider ultrasound scan/CT AP to confirm collection/active bleeding. If unstable, will likely need to go to theatre. In that case, liaise with theatre co-ordinator, porters, blood bank and anaesthetist and consent patient if you are able to.<br>• Consider O negative blood if unstable. | /5 |
| Appropriate management of Mrs D:<br>• Do not disclose any information.<br>• State GMC guidelines on confidentiality and good medical practice.<br>• Confidentiality is an essential part of the doctor-patient relationship<br>• Doctors are under both ethical and legal duties to protect patients' personal information. | /5 |
| Appropriate management of Ms E:<br>• Impression: Post-operative pain, not on any analgesia, PCA down.<br>• Management: Ask FY1 to assess and prescribe analgesia and insert cannula. | /5 |
| Total | /30 |

# CLINICAL STATION 2

You are the FY2 on-call and have received the following bleeps within a 5 minute period. Please read through the scenarios below and then discuss with the examiner about how you will prioritise the scenarios below. The General Surgical Registrar, Orthopaedic Registrar, Gynaecology Registrar and FY1 can be contacted.

A. 78-Year-old, Mr A confused day 2 following Neck of Femur fracture. Observations: Heart rate 120, temperature 38, respiratory rate 25, blood pressure 100/60. Sats 92% air.

B. 28-year-old, Ms B with right iliac fossa pain in A&E. Observations: Heart rate 110, temperature 38, respiratory rate 18, oxygen saturations 98%, blood pressure 98/66.

C. Patient waiting on discharge summary and threatening to self-discharge.

D. The haematology consultant asks about his mother's CT results which shows metastasis.

E. 30-year-old, Ms E, admitted with early miscarriage (confirmed on USS) and has a background history of mental health problems. Observations: Heart rate 85, Temperature 37, Respiratory rate 18, Oxygen saturations 100%, blood pressure 120/80.

# CLINICAL STATION 2 - MARK SCHEME

| | |
|---|---|
| Rapid assessment and prioritisation (ABECD) | /5 |
| Appropriate management of Mr A:<br>• Observations: Heart rate 120, temperature 38, respiratory rate 25, blood pressure 100/60. Sats 92% air.<br>• Investigations: Urine dipstick, CXR, FBC/U&E/CRP<br>• Impression: UNSTABLE, see First. Hospital Acquired Pneumonia<br>• Management: Full assessment, cardiorespiratory. (productive cough, chest reduced air entry right side), CNS, GI, ENT, Urogenital. To do full septic screen (ABG/lactate, bloods, blood cultures, mid-stream urine, sputum culture, intravenous access, intravenous fluids). Confirm allergy status and commence IV antibiotics based on local protocol. If patient spikes temperature again, liaise with microbiologist/inform seniors.<br>• Other causes of confusion in elderly. Sepsis, Urinary Retention, Hypoxia (?PE), TIA, Hypoglycaemia, Drug misuse, Alcohol withdrawal. | /5 |
| Appropriate management of B:<br>• Observations: Heart rate 110, temperature 38, respiratory rate 18, oxygen saturations 98%, blood pressure 98/66.<br>• Investigations: Urine dip/pregnancy test, FBC/U&E/CRP etc<br>• Impression: Likely appendicitis, suspected sepsis.<br>• Management: Perform full septic screen. Obtain senior input from general surgical registrar. | /5 |
| Appropriate management of C:<br>• Ask FY1, if available to complete the discharge Summary.<br>• If no other people available, inform ward sister, apologise to the patient, that the doctor is currently busy, attending to an unwell patient and will complete it as soon as possible.<br>• If patient is adamant to go, must sign self-discharge form.<br>• Discharge summary will be posted in due course. | /5 |
| Appropriate management of D:<br><br>Do not disclose any information.<br>• State GMC guidelines on confidentiality and good medical practice.<br>• Confidentiality is an essential part of the doctor-patient relationship<br>• Doctors are under both ethical and legal duties to protect patients' personal information.<br>• Apologise to the son and express you can-not breach patient confidentiality.<br>• The son can directly speak to his mother regarding the results of her investigations.<br>• With patient's consent, he can attend the morning ward round to learn about his mother's progress.<br>• If you are not able to speak to the son directly, delegate the above task to the ward sister. | /5 |

| | |
|---|---|
| Appropriate management of Ms E:<br>• Observations: Stable, afebrile.<br>• Impression: Complete Miscarriage.<br>• Management: physical examination including abdominal and speculum<br>• Assess for 'red flag' signs for severe maternal illness and if any "red flag" request an urgent senior psychiatric assessment + admit.<br>• New thoughts or acts of violent self-harm<br>• Rapidly changing mental state,<br>• Pervasive guilt or hopelessness,<br>• Evidence of psychosis. | /5 |
| Total | /30 |

# CLINICAL STATION 3

You have received the following bleeps within a 5 minute period. Please read through the scenarios below and then discuss with the examiner about how you will prioritise the scenarios below. The Medical Registrar, Orthopaedic Registrar, Gynaecology Registrar and FY1 can be contacted.

A. 77-year-old, Mrs A on the medical ward with post-menopausal bleeding. Observations: Heart rate 80, blood pressure 142/88, afebrile.

B. 77-year-old, Mr B who is feeling unwell and short of breath, 3 days post Total Hip Replacement. Observations: Blood pressure 100/70, heart rate 120, oxygen saturations 88% on air, respiratory rate 22, afebrile.

C. 22-year-old, Ms C in A&E with a vulval haematoma following a horse riding accident. Observations: Heart rate 88, blood pressure 120/80, afebrile.

D. 32-year-old, Ms D in A&E who is 14 weeks pregnant with a history of asthma and is complaining of shortness of breath. Observations: Respiratory rate 28, oxygen saturations 91%, heart rate 110, blood pressure 130/88.

E. 79-year-old, Mr E uncomfortable, not opened his bowels for 4 days. Observation is stable, Afebrile.

# CLINICAL STATION 3 - MARK SCHEME

| | |
|---|---|
| Rapid assessment and prioritisation (BDCEA) | /5 |
| Appropriate management of Ms A:<br>• Investigations: Haemoglobin 110g/L, not on warfarin.<br>• Impression: Post-menopausal bleeding, but stable.<br>• Management: Ask medical team to arrange transvaginal ultrasound and gynaecology follow up as target (cancer pathway).<br>• State I Will review when free or handover the incoming on call | /5 |
| Appropriate management of Mr B:<br>• Other bedside information: Good urine output.<br>• Investigations: Not had any yet.<br>• Impression: Pulmonary embolism<br>• Management: UNSTABLE, see FIRST.<br>• Investigations: Electrocardiogram, ABG, Bloods - including D-dimer, CXR. CTPA/V/Q scan<br>• Treatment: Oxygen, intravenous access, inform senior and medical team. Start treatment dose low molecular weight heparin pending results of scan. | /5 |
| Appropriate management of Ms C:<br>• Other information: Not actively bleeding.<br>• Investigations: Urine dipstick and urinary pregnancy test negative<br>• Management: Take bloods and give analgesia and icepack whilst awaiting review). | /5 |
| Appropriate management of Ms D:<br>• Impression: Acute exacerbation of asthma. PE may need to be ruled out - unwell.<br>• Management: Explain acute management of asthma safe in pregnancy. High flow O2, Salbutamol Nebuliser, Prednisolone. Bloods FBC, CRP and ABG. ECG, if require chest x-ray benefits outweigh risks of radiation. | /5 |
| Appropriate management of Mr E:<br>• Other information: No vomiting, eating and drinking well.<br>• On codeine phosphate following knee replacement.<br>• Impression: Likely constipation,<br>• Management: will need an abdominal x-ray, FY1 to assess and prescribe lactulose, if no FY1, will review in due course. | /5 |
| Total | /30 |

# CLINICAL STATION 4

You have received the following bleeps within a 5 minute period. Please read through the scenarios below and then discuss with the examiner about how you will prioritise the scenarios below. The General Surgical Registrar, Orthopaedic Registrar, Gynaecology Registrar and FY1 can be contacted.

A. A cannula required on the ward for a patient with gastroenteritis. Observations stable. Urine dip, +3 ketones

B. 23-year-old, Ms B, presenting to A&E with left iliac fossa pain. Observations: HR 120, BP 93/56, Temp 36.6, RR 18, Sats 98%

C. 30-year-old, Ms C, who is 24 weeks pregnant with back pain and rigors. Observations: Temperature 38, blood pressure 130/84, heart rate 88. Investigations: Urine dipstick: leucocytes 3+ nitrites + protein +.

D. 65-year-old, Mrs D, in the acute assessment unit with an abdominal mass. Observations stable, afebrile

E. Patient on medical ward needing INR level done, before given warfarin.

# CLINICAL STATION 4 - MARK SCHEME

| | |
|---|---|
| Rapid assessment and prioritisation (BCEAD) | /5 |
| Appropriate management of Ms A:<br>• Impression- Dehydration<br>• Management: Ask FY1 to cannulate. FY1 to prescribe iv fluids. | /5 |
| Appropriate management of Ms B:<br>• Investigation. Urine dipstick (negative) and urine pregnancy test (positive). Organise an urgent ultrasound scan if stable. Blood test (full blood count, renal function and electrolytes, CRP, group and save).<br>• Management: Obtain intravenous access, 2 large bore cannulae and fluid resuscitate, VBG. Cross match 4-6 units of blood.<br>• Inform Gynaecology registrar/consultant.<br>Will likely need to go to theatre. (inform anaesthetist, porters, theatre co-ordinator)<br>• Impression: Likely raptured ectopic pregnancy.<br>• Consent if able. Laparoscopy +- salpingotomy +- salpingectomy, risk of Bleeding, Infection. Damage to nearby structures (bladder, bowel, ureters, blood vessels), Thromboembolic disease, Anaesthetic risks,<br>• If salpingotomy, will need further monitoring and rarely further procedure.<br>• Other procedures: blood transfusion, laparotomy, repair of any damage, oophorectomy. | /5 |
| Appropriate management of Ms C:<br>• Investigations: Urine dipstick: leucocytes 3+ nitrites + protein +.<br>• Impression: Likely pyelonephritis.<br>• Management: If FY1 is available, can ask them to see assess and prescribe intravenous fluids, intravenous antibiotics, analgesia, send of bloods and septic screen and inform obstetric/medical registrar. Consider USS renal. | /5 |
| Appropriate management of Ms D:<br>• Management: Ask for tumour markers, CA125, CA119, medical team to arrange target (two week wait appointment, cancer pathway).<br>• Arrange transvaginal ultrasound and gynaecology outpatient follow up.<br>• You will review once you are free, if not handover to oncoming team. | /5 |
| Appropriate management of Ms E:<br>• Management: Ask FY1/Site nurse practitioner to perform INR | /5 |
| Total | /30 |

# CLINICAL STATION 5

You have received the following bleeps within a 5 minute period. Please read through the scenarios below and then discuss with the examiner about how you will prioritise the scenarios below. The General Surgical Registrar, Orthopaedic Registrar, Gynaecology Registrar and FY1 can be contacted.

A. 45 year old male on surgical ward, reporting haematemesis. Observations: HR 120, BP 90/40, Temp 36.1, RR 24, Sats 96% RA

B. 23 year old female on orthopaedic ward having blood transfusion post-op, reporting a fever. Observations: BP 120/80, 90bpm, 100% RA, RR18, T38.0

C. 88 year old female with pain after hip replacement. Observations: BP 130/80, 80bpm, 98% on RA, RR17, T37.2

D. Son of patient C calls you requesting an update on his mother.

# CLINICAL STATION 5 - MARK SCHEME

| | |
|---|---|
| Rapid assessment and prioritisation (ABCD) | /5 |
| Appropriate management of Ms A:<br>• Establishes this is most unwell patient and should be prioritised.<br>• Investigations: FBC, U&Es, LFTs, Clotting, VBG, G&S. CXR (pneumoperitoneum)<br>• Impression- Upper GI bleed (differentials: peptic ulcer perforation, Mallory-Weiss Tear, Variceal bleed)<br>• Management: Full A-E assessment: including administering O2, inserting 2 large bore cannulas and taking bloods, Cross match 2-4 units, give stat IV fluids. Monitor urine output and commence fluid balance chart.<br>• As they are harm-dynamically unstable with ongoing bleeding, can consider major haemorrhage protocol and give O- blood.<br>• Escalate to general surgical registrar to review patient, and consideration of taking to theatre. | /5 |
| Appropriate management of Ms B:<br>• Patient is haemodynamically stable. As you will be resuscitating patient A, ask nurse to stop the transfusion immediately until you arrive. They can put out 2222 call if any concerning features e.g. hypoxia/hypotension<br>• Impression: Febrile non-haemolytic reaction (Differentials: bacterial contamination, acute haemolytic transfusion reaction, anaphylaxis, TRALI)<br>• Investigation: if you suspect haemolysis, you can send off FBC/LDH/Bilirubin/Clotting etc, blood cultures if you suspect bacterial contamination<br>• Management: A-E assessment including checking for signs of anaphylaxis (dyspnoea, stridor, hypoxia, hypotension). If temperature ≥ 38.0 or rise of 1-2°C, itching/rash only - continue with transfusion. Treat symptoms i.e. Chlorphenamine. Monitor closely for any deterioration. | /5 |
| Appropriate management of Ms C:<br>• Send FY1 to review patient. Give them advice on what to look for: exclude common post-op complications including DVT, infection, bleeding.<br>• Ensure analgesia is appropriate as per analgesia ladder<br>• Impression: Likely post-op pain<br>• Management: Prescribe appropriate analgesia as per analgesia ladder. Obtain handover from FY1 afterwards. | /5 |
| Appropriate management of son of patient C:<br>• As FY1 is reviewing Ms C, they can update the son afterwards. Ensure that you/FY1 has patient's permission to provide their son with information and what they would like disclosed. | /5 |
| Total | /25 |

# CLINICAL STATION 6

You are the FY2 on call and have received the following bleeps within a 5 minute period. Please read through the scenarios below and then discuss with the examiner about how you will prioritise the scenarios below. The Medical Registrar, Orthopaedic Registrar, Gynaecology Registrar and FY1 can be contacted.

A. 70-year-old Mrs A, on the orthopedic ward four days following a hip operation, complaining of acute onset chest pain. Observations: Blood pressure 95/60, heart rate 120, oxygen saturations 88% on air, respiratory rate 25, afebrile

B. 50-year-old Mr B, on the surgical ward, is post-op following a colectomy, and his PCA has been stopped and he is screaming in pain. Observations: Heart rate 120, blood pressure 72/48, temperature 36, respiratory rate 22, oxygen saturations 100 percent on air. Low urine output.

C. 80-year-old, Mrs C, admitted to the ward awaiting elective total hip replacement is now appearing confused. Observations: Heart rate 90, blood pressure 120/80, respiratory rate 18, T38.1, Oxygen saturations 100% on air.

D. 35-year-old Ms D contacts the ward requesting to know their HIV result.

# CLINICAL STATION 6 - MARK SCHEME

| | |
|---|---|
| Rapid assessment and prioritisation (ABCD) | /5 |
| Appropriate management of Ms A:<br>• Impression: Pulmonary embolism. Differentials: Myocardial infarction<br>• Management: UNSTABLE, see FIRST.<br>• Investigations: Electrocardiogram, ABG, Bloods - FBC/U&E/Clotting/D-dimer, CXR. CTPA/V/Q scan<br>• Treatment: Oxygen, intravenous access, inform senior and medical team. Start treatment dose low molecular weight heparin pending results of scan +/- consideration of thrombolysis | /10 |
| Appropriate management of Mrs B:<br>• Impression: UNSTABLE. Post-operative bleed.<br>• Management – Inform seniors/operating team and anaesthetist. Ensure two large bore cannulae, intravenous fluids, oxygen, bloods including full blood count, group and save and venous blood gas for immediate haemoglobin. Cross match 4 units.<br>• Blood tests/gas to look for signs of anaemia secondary to haemorrhage, raised lactate and metabolic acidosis secondary to heamorrhagic shock/sepsis.<br>• If stabilises, consider ultrasound scan/CT AP to confirm collection/active bleeding. If unstable, will likely need to go to theatre. In that case, liaise with theatre co-ordinator, porters, blood bank and anaesthetist and consent patient if you are able to.<br>• Consider O negative blood if unstable. | /10 |
| Appropriate management of Mr C:<br>• Investigations: Urine dip, send MSU/CXR, bloods; FBC, U&E, CRP<br>• Impression: Infection - delirium<br>• Management: Full assessment, cardiorespiratory, CNS, GI, ENT, Urogenital. Confirm allergy status, and commence antibiotics based on local protocol. IV access and IV fluids. If patient spikes temperature, to do full septic screen and liaise with microbiologist/inform seniors.<br>• Other causes of confusion in elderly. Sepsis, Urinary Retention, Hypoxia (?PE), TIA, Hypoglycaemia, Drug misuse, Alcohol withdrawal. | /5 |
| Appropriate management of Mr D:<br>• Do not disclose any information over the phone.<br>• State GMC guidelines on confidentiality and good medical practice.<br>• Confidentiality is an essential part of the doctor-patient relationship<br>• Doctors are under both ethical and legal duties to protect patients' personal information.<br>• Arrange for patient to come in to receive the results | /5 |
| Total | /35 |

# CLINICAL STATION 7

You are the FY2 on call and have received the following bleeps within a 5 minute period. Please read through the scenarios below and then discuss with the examiner about how you will prioritise the scenarios below. The Medical Registrar, Orthopaedic Registrar, Gynaecology Registrar and FY1 can be contacted.

A. 55-year-old Mrs A, on the medical ward receiving treatment for pneumonia, found to have abdominal mass on examination. Observations: Blood pressure 120/80, heart rate 90, oxygen saturations 99% on air, respiratory rate 19, afebrile.

B. 45-year-old Mr B on surgical ward, reporting large haematemesis. Observations: HR 120, BP 90/40, Temp 36.1, RR 24, Sats 96% RA

C. 30-year-old Mrs C on the gynaecology ward has had ERPC for miscarriage. She is reporting pain and analgesia needs to be prescribed. Observations: HR 80, BP 120/80, Temp 36.1, RR 18, Sats 99% RA

D. Husband of Mrs C calling the ward to receive an update about her.

E. 40-year-old Mrs D receiving a blood transfusion for anaemia secondary to menorrhagia, feeling feverish and flushed. Observations: T38.1, BP 120/80, HR 90bpm, RR 19, Sats 100% RA.

# CLINICAL STATION 7 - MARK SCHEME

| | |
|---|---|
| Rapid assessment and prioritisation (BECAD) | /5 |
| Appropriate management of Mrs A:<br>• Impression: STABLE. Multiple differentials: including ovarian cancer, fibroids - as per NICE guidelines, refer women urgently if physical examination identifies ascites and/or pelvic or abdominal mass (which is not obviously uterine fibroids)<br>• Management: Needs full history and examination to narrow down differentials + explore possibility of malignancy<br>• Investigations: Bloods - FBC/U&E/LFTs, tumour markers including CA-125, USS Abdomen<br>• Treatment: Refer urgently under 2ww pathway | /5 |
| Appropriate management of Mrs B:<br>• Establishes this is most unwell patient and should be prioritised.<br>• Investigations: FBC, U&Es, LFTs, Clotting, VBG, G&S. CXR (pneumoperitoneum)<br>• Impression- Upper GI bleed, UNSTABLE (differentials: peptic ulcer perforation, Mallory-Weiss Tear, Variceal bleed)<br>• Management: Full A-E assessment: including administering O2, inserting 2 large bore cannulas and taking bloods, Cross match 2-4 units, give stat IV fluids. Monitor urine output and commence fluid balance chart.<br>• As they are harm-dynamically unstable with ongoing bleeding, can consider major haemorrhage protocol and give O- blood.<br>• Escalate to general surgical registrar to review patient, and consideration of taking to theatre. | /5 |
| Appropriate management of Mrs C:<br>• Send FY1 to review patient.<br>• Ensure analgesia is appropriate as per analgesia ladder<br>• Impression: Likely post-op pain<br>• Management: Prescribe appropriate analgesia as per analgesia ladder. Obtain handover from FY1 afterwards. | /5 |
| Appropriate management of Mrs C's husband:<br>• Update only with Mrs C's permission - after confirming with her what she information we can pass on to her husband.<br>• State GMC guidelines on confidentiality and good medical practice.<br>• Confidentiality is an essential part of the doctor-patient relationship<br>• Doctors are under both ethical and legal duties to protect patients' personal information. | /5 |

| | |
|---|---|
| Appropriate management of Mrs D:<br>• Patient is haemodynamically stable. As you will be resuscitating patient B, ask nurse to stop the transfusion immediately until you arrive. They can put out 2222 call if any concerning features e.g. hypoxia/ hypotension<br>• Impression: Febrile non-haemolytic reaction (Differentials: bacterial contamination, acute haemolytic transfusion reaction, anaphylaxis, TRALI)<br>• Investigation: if you suspect haemolysis, you can send off FBC/LDH/ Bilirubin/Clotting etc, blood cultures if you suspect bacterial contamination<br>• Management: A-E assessment including checking for signs of anaphylaxis (dyspnoea, stridor, hypoxia, hypotension). If temperature ≥ 38.0 or rise of 1-2°C, itching/rash only - continue with transfusion. Treat symptoms i.e. Chlorphenamine. Monitor closely for any deterioration. | /5 |
| Total | /30 |

# CLINICAL STATION 8

You are the FY2 on call and have received the following bleeps within a 5 minute period. Please read through the scenarios below and then discuss with the examiner about how you will prioritise the scenarios below. The Medical Registrar, Orthopaedic Registrar, Urology Registrar and FY1 can be contacted.

A. 80-year-old, Mrs C, admitted to the ward awaiting elective total hip replacement and is appearing confused. Observations: Heart rate 90, blood pressure 120/80, respiratory rate 18, T38.1, Oxygen saturations 100% on air.

B. 45-year-old Mr B arriving in A&E with significant RIF pain. Observations: HR 120, BP 90/40, Temp 38.5, RR 24, Sats 96% RA

C. 30-year-old Mrs C on the surgical ward with suspected renal stones. She is reporting worsening pain and vomiting. Observations: HR 110, BP 120/80, Temp 36.1, RR 18, Sats 99% RA

D. 35-year-old Mr D contacts the ward requesting to know their HIV result.

# CLINICAL STATION 8 - MARK SCHEME

| | |
|---|---|
| Rapid assessment and prioritisation (BCAD) | /5 |
| Appropriate management of Mrs A:<br>• Investigations: Urine dip, send MSU/CXR, bloods; FBC, U&E, CRP<br>• Impression: Infection - delirium<br>• Management: Full assessment, cardiorespiratory, CNS, GI, ENT, Uro-genital. Confirm allergy status, and commence antibiotics based on local protocol. IV access and IV fluids. If patient spikes temperature, to do full septic screen and liaise with microbiologist/inform seniors.<br>• Other causes of confusion in elderly. Sepsis, Urinary Retention, Hypoxia (?PE), TIA, Hypoglycaemia, Drug misuse, Alcohol withdrawal. | /5 |
| Appropriate management of Mrs B:<br>• Establishes this is most unwell patient and should be prioritised.<br>• Investigations: FBC, U&Es, LFTs, Clotting, VBG, G&S. CXR (pneumoperitoneum)<br>• Impression- Perforated appendix, UNSTABLE<br>• Management: Full A-E assessment: including administering O2, inserting 2 large bore cannulas and taking bloods, give stat IV fluids and IV Abx. Monitor urine output and commence fluid balance chart.<br>• Need to transfer to theatre urgently for appendectomy<br>• Escalate to general surgical registrar to review patient | /10 |
| Appropriate management of Mrs C:<br>• Impression: Renal stones, need to exclude urinary tract obstruction/ infection<br>• Investigations: FBC/U&Es/VBG/CRP, Bladder scan to look for retention, CTKUB to look for signs of obstruction<br>• Management: Prescribe appropriate analgesia as per analgesia ladder. Escalate to urology registrar to review if obstruction seen | /5 |
| Appropriate management of Mr D:<br>• Do not disclose any information over the phone.<br>• State GMC guidelines on confidentiality and good medical practice.<br>• Confidentiality is an essential part of the doctor-patient relationship<br>• Doctors are under both ethical and legal duties to protect patients' personal information.<br>• Arrange for patient to come in to receive the results | /5 |
| Total | /30 |

# CLINICAL STATION 9

You are the FY2 on call and have received the following bleeps within a 5 minute period. Please read through the scenarios below and then discuss with the examiner about how you will prioritise the scenarios below. The General Surgical Registrar, Orthopaedic Registrar, Gynaecology Registrar and FY1 can be contacted.

A. 32-year-old, Mrs A, is 8/40 and presenting to A&E with vomiting and not tolerating oral intake for 24h. Observations: Heart rate 90, blood pressure 120/80, respiratory rate 18, T37, Oxygen saturations 100% on air.

B. The mother of patient A has telephoned the ward and wants to speak to you as she is unhappy about the care A has received since being there.

C. 50-year-old Mr B, on the surgical ward, is post-op following a colectomy, and he is experiencing worsening pain. Observations: Heart rate 120, blood pressure 72/48, temperature 36, respiratory rate 22, oxygen saturations 100 percent on air.

D. 70-year-old Mrs D on the geriatric ward is reporting an extremely painful R leg - the nurse feels it is cold to touch and cannot palpate pulses. Heart rate 110, blood pressure 120/80, respiratory rate 18, T37, Oxygen saturations 100% on air.

# CLINICAL STATION 9 - MARK SCHEME

| | |
|---|---|
| Rapid assessment and prioritisation (CDAB) | /5 |
| Appropriate management of Mrs A:<br>• Investigations: Urine dip (for ketones), send MSU, bloods; FBC/U&E, BM/LFTs (exclude liver disease causes e.g. hepatitis or gallstones), Amylase (exclude pancreatitis)<br>• Impression: Hyperemesis Gravidarum, differentials: Nausea and vomiting in pregnancy, Gastroenteritis<br>• Management: As she is unable to tolerate oral intake - admit, IV fluids, anti-emetics (e.g. cyclizine, metoclopramide, ondansetron) and monitor ketonuria<br>• USS to confirm viable intrauterine pregnancy and exclude multiple pregnancy and trophoblastic disease | /5 |
| Appropriate management of Mrs A's mother:<br>• State GMC guidelines on confidentiality and good medical practice.<br>• Confidentiality is an essential part of the doctor-patient relationship<br>• Doctors are under both ethical and legal duties to protect patients' personal information.<br>• With Mrs A's permission you can update the mother and only disclose information that she is happy to be shared about the care. Offer PALS. | /5 |
| Appropriate management of Mrs C:<br>• Impression: UNSTABLE. Post-operative bleed. First priority<br>• Management – Inform seniors/operating team and anaesthetist. Ensure two large bore cannulae, intravenous fluids, oxygen, bloods including full blood count, group and save and venous blood gas for immediate haemoglobin. Cross match 4 units.<br>• Blood tests/gas to look for signs of anaemia secondary to haemorrhage, raised lactate and metabolic acidosis secondary to heamorrhagic shock/sepsis.<br>• If stabilises, consider ultrasound scan/CT AP to confirm collection/ active bleeding. If unstable, will likely need to go to theatre. In that case, liaise with theatre co-ordinator, porters, blood bank and anaesthetist and consent patient if you are able to.<br>• Consider O negative blood if unstable. | /10 |
| Appropriate management of Mrs D:<br>• Impression: Acute limb ischaemia. Differentials: DVT, compartment syndrome<br>• Management - Assessment for signs of ALI - 6Ps (pain, pallor, paraesthesia, paralysis, perishingly cold, pulselessness) and risk factors. ECG (AF/cardiac arrhythmias that could be source of embolus), Bloods - FBC/U&E/CK/Clotting/G&S. Imaging: MR/CT angiogram<br>• Treatment: Analgesia, oxygen, IV Heparin, IV fluids (patient's with ALI can be dehydrated). Urgent referral to vascular surgery for revascularisation. | /5 |
| Total | /30 |

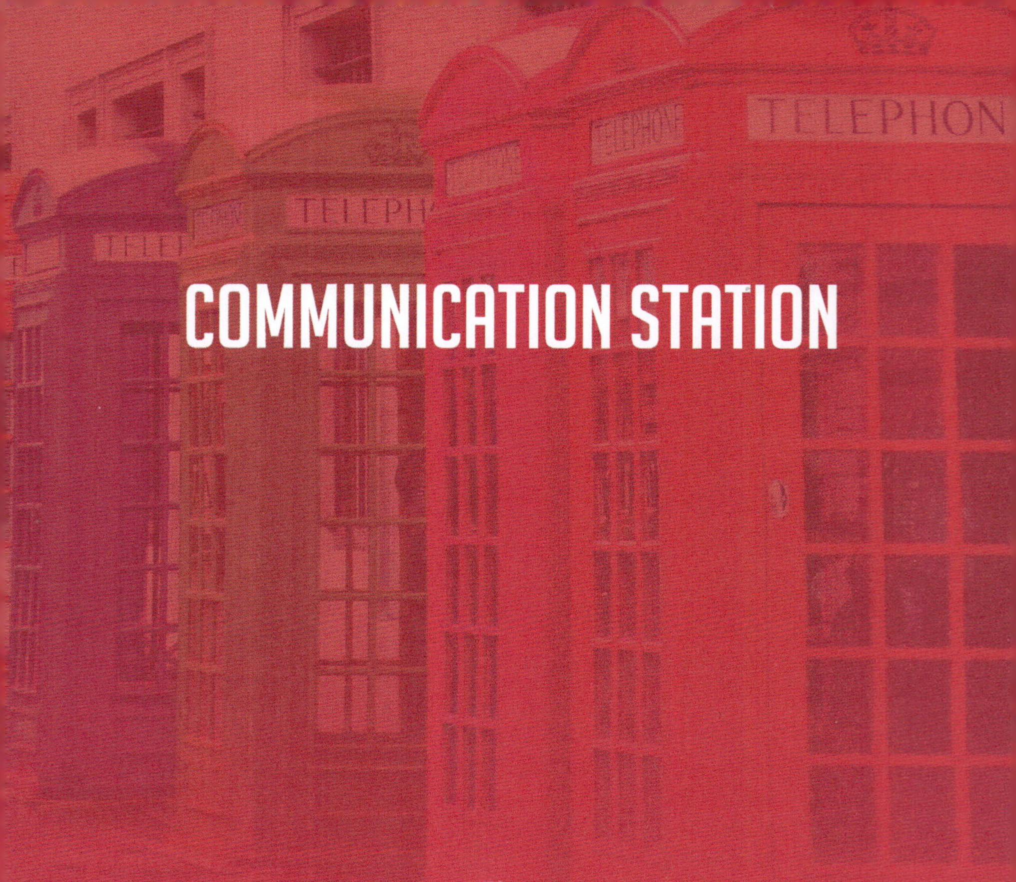


# COMMUNICATION STATION

OBSTETRICS AND GYNAECOLOGY ST1 INTERVIEW BOOK

obsandgynae.net

# COMMUNICATION STATION

Although this is named the "communication station", do not be fooled. It tests a combination of clinical and communication skills.

- General advice:
  - Scenarios are designed to be realistic, therefore remain calm and act as you would in reality – If you were called to see this patient, what would you do?
  - Would you want to know their observations? If the answer is yes, then ask for them.
    e.g. "We are just going to put a small monitor on your finger and a blood pressure cuff on your arm just to check a few of your measurements."
  - Would you want an electrocardiogram (ECG)?
    e.g. "We are going to put some leads on your chest to measure the activity of your heart."
  - Scenarios are very repetitive – practice previous scenarios!
  - Use non-medical terminology.
  - Introduce yourself and your role at the start of the consultation and offer follow-up at the end.
  - Give information in bite-sized pieces and check for understanding.

# COMMON SCENARIOS

- Anaemia due to menorrhagia history/postnatally and consenting for a blood transfusion
- Pulmonary Embolism followed by management of angry patient
- Ectopic pregnancy history and consent for surgery
- Incomplete miscarriage and consent for Surgical Management of Miscarriage
- Appendicitis followed by management of angry patient
- Cancelled hysterectomy due to lung nodule followed by management of angry patient

# PULMONARY EMBOLISM

### HISTORY
Ensure you take a full history of the pain (use SOCRATES mnemonic). Ask about associated symptoms (including cough, fever, calf pain, shortness of breath, palpitations, dizziness), risk factors for pulmonary embolism (recent travel/surgery, immobilisation, fractured bones, use of combined oral contraceptive pill, personal or family history, smoker).

### EXAMINATION
Ask for observations, perform a cardiac/respiratory exam and examine calves.

### INVESTIGATIONS
Bloods (full blood count, C-reactive protein, D-dimer), arterial blood gas, electrocardiogram (ECG), chest x-ray, ventilation perfusion scan (V/Q scan)/CT pulmonary angiogram (CTPA).

### OXYGEN
In the history, if the patient states that they are short of breath, say "I am just going to put an oxygen mask on you to help you breathe."

### MANAGEMENT
Ask if they want anyone in the room when you explain the diagnosis and further management. Explain that the shortness of breath may be due to a clot in the lungs. You will start them on a blood thinning injection to prevent spread of any clot until further imaging.

- Patient may ask, "Will I be okay Doctor?"
  - Example answer: It's a good thing you came into hospital and we have picked this up early. If picked up early like in your case, and treated properly, it is unlikely to cause any significant long term problems. However, we do need to keep you in hospital and keep a close eye on you at the moment.

# PULMONARY EMBOLISM STATION (2) - ANGRY PATIENT

"You are a different doctor. The patient comes to see you as they are upset about being sent home without advice regarding INR monitoring on warfarin. This led to them having a significant nose bleed."

**APOLOGISE**

- Listen. Allow the patient time to express their concerns.
- Apologise for the distress caused.

**INVESTIGATE**

- Plan to obtain notes and review these with a senior to assess how care could have been improved.
- Put in an incident report, which goes to the management team who will investigate the case.
- Consider organising teaching or bringing up the issue at the next departmental meeting to bring about awareness and prevent recurrence.
- Offer the patient details of Patient Advice and Liaison Service (PALS) if they want to put it an official complaint.

**FOLLOW UP**

- Offer the patient a follow up meeting to discuss the outcome of any investigation.
- Is there anything else we can do to help you?

**GENERAL MEDICAL CARE**

- How is the patient otherwise? How is their recovery and how are their symptoms?
- If complaint is about lack of explanation regarding condition and management, explain this to them and provide a leaflet.

# ANGRY PATIENT

**USEFUL PHRASES**

- "I apologise for the distress this has caused you. It is important that we investigate it thoroughly so that we can take steps to prevent it happening in the future."
- "Doctors and nurses would never intentionally give suboptimal care. I'm sure my colleague would appreciate this feedback and I will definitely pass it along to him/her."
- "I'm sorry you feel like you have not been given the information you need."

# ANAEMIA DUE TO MENORRHAGIA

## HISTORY

- History of menorrhagia (need for double protection, any clots, flooding).
- Symptoms of anaemia (shortness of breath, dizziness, fatigue).
- Effect on quality of life.
- Menstrual cycle (age at menarche, regularity of cycles, how long bleeds are, intermenstrual/postcoital bleeding, dysmenorrhoea, dyspareunia).
- Gynaecological history (smear results, contraception, any previous sexually transmitted infections).
- Obstetric history (parity and outcome of any pregnancies).
- Exclude other potential sources of bleeding.
  1. History of presenting complaint (any rectal bleeding, malaena, weight loss, night sweats or haemoptysis which could suggest gastrointestinal, respiratory or malignant cause).
  2. Medication history (use of steroids/non-steroidal anti inflammatory drug could predispose to peptic ulcer).
  3. Recent surgery (post-operative bleed).
  4. Social history (alcohol and cirrhosis suggestive of variceal bleed).

## EXAMINATION

- Ask for observations and perform a full examination. You may then be told that relevant findings include a heart rate of 120 and a palpable fibroid uterus.

# ANAEMIA DUE TO MENORRHAGIA

## COUNSELING FOR BLOOD TRANSFUSION

- Counsel regarding
  1. Type of blood products
  2. Indication for transfusion
  3. Benefits and risks
  4. Possible alternatives (e.g. iron infusion)
  5. How transfusion is administered
- Inform patient that following a blood transfusion they can no longer be a donor.
- Give written information.
- Check if patient needs time to consider/any further information.

## RISKS OF BLOOD TRANSFUSION

- Viral Infections
  - HIV: 1 in 6 million
  - Hepatitis: 1 in 1 million
  - Hep C: 1 in 72 million
- Allergic or immune reaction: common
- Anaphylaxis/immune reaction: serious but rare
- Development of antibodies

## EXAMPLE ANSWER

- The reason you are feeling tired and short of breath is because you have a low red blood count. We suspect this is because of the heavy bleeding you have been having.
- We would recommend a blood transfusion, where we put a drip into your arm and replace those blood cells, which will make you feel better.
- Blood transfusions are fairly common. The risk of serious side effects is low. There is a small risk of infection, but all blood donors are carefully selected and tested for infections to ensure blood donated is as safe as possible. The risk of hepatitis or HIV is less than 1 in a million.

- Some people who have a blood transfusion can have an allergic reaction. This is usually just a little bit of itching and we can give you tablets to help with that. Rarely, you could have a severe allergic reaction.
- There is a risk of your body reacting to the blood products by producing antibodies. Antibodies are small protein molecules that circulate in the blood and recognise certain molecules as foreign. This may make it more difficult to obtain compatible blood if you require transfusion in the future.
- You will be regularly monitored whilst having the blood transfusion and immediately after it. This includes checking your blood pressure, heart rate and pulse. If you develop any signs of having a reaction, we would stop the transfusion straight away and start any necessary treatment.

**ALTERNATIVES**

- Iron tablets – Iron is a component of red blood cells. Iron tablets slowly increase blood levels over the next six to eight weeks. Side effects include constipation and vomiting.
- Iron infusion – Increases iron levels over 2-3 weeks. Small risk of allergic reaction.
- Ask if they have any questions and if there is anything else you can advise them about to help make their decision.
- Give a leaflet.

# PELVIC INFLAMMATORY DISEASE

## HISTORY

- "I will need to ask you some personal questions. Everything you say is confidential and any information you provide will help to work out what is causing your pain so we can treat you effectively."
- If any discharge, ask about colour, itchiness, odour.
- Any pain or irregular bleeding?
- When was her last sexual intercourse? Regular or casual partner? Male or female? Type of sex?
- Any history of sexually transmitted infections?
- Contraception use?
- Previous pregnancies?

## EXAMINATION

- "I am going to put a probe on your finger and a cuff around your arm to get some basic measurements. We will also measure your temperature. I am then going to feel your tummy and do an internal examination and take some infection swabs. Would this be okay? Nurse Emma will be here as a chaperone and we will lock the door to ensure your privacy."

## INVESTIGATIONS

- "We need to do some blood tests to look at your infection markers. Would that be okay? We also need to test your urine for infection and to test for a pregnancy. We will also organise a ultrasound scan of the tummy."

## DIAGNOSIS AND MANAGEMENT

- Say that you are going to explain the diagnosis and management. Does she want anyone in the room with them whilst you go through it?
- "The pain you are having is most likely due to an infection in the womb and tubes. We call this pelvic inflammatory disease."

# PELVIC INFLAMMATORY DISEASE

- "The infection is treated by giving you a course of antibiotics for 14 days. It is very important that you complete the course even if you are feeling better as if you stop part way through the course, the infection can recur, resulting in complications."
- "As this may be due to a sexually transmitted infection, it is important that you refrain from sexual intercourse or use barrier contraception such as condoms whilst you are on treatment. You should attend a sexual health clinic and have a sexual health screen after the treatment is complete, to ensure that the infection has cleared."
- "It is also important that your partner is treated regardless of what screening shows. Most males are asymptomatic and screening only picks up about half of cases. If any partners have the infection and it is not treated, the infection will pass back and forth."
- "We advise that you inform any partners that you have had in the last six months, so that they can receive the appropriate treatment and prevent long-term complications. The sexual health clinic can do this for you if you prefer."

**LONG TERM COUNSELING**

- "There are some potential long term consequences of this condition. These risks increase with recurrent episodes of this condition, therefore, it is important you take steps from preventing a recurrence."
- "These complications include long term pain, difficulty getting pregnant and pregnancies occurring outside the womb and in one of the tubes known as ectopic pregnancies."
- "To prevent this happening again, it is important to use condoms. It is important to know that whilst other forms of contraception prevent pregnancies, they do not prevent sexually transmitted infections. It is also important to have regular sexual health checks if you have a new partner or symptoms such as abnormal vaginal discharge or pain in your tummy."

# APPENDICITIS

You are the A&E SHO reviewing a 34 year old lady who has presented with right iliac fossa pain, fevers and vomiting. She has been waiting in A&E for the last 4 hours therefore is about to breech the 4 hour wait protocol. Please take a history and advise the patient regarding further management options.

**PART 2 OF STATION –**

- Option 1- You're seeing the patient after 48-72 hours. She has had an appendicectomy and is clinically better. However, she has some concerns about the level of care (delay in surgical review/delay in antibiotics)
- Option 2 – She was discharged after your review as it was felt that she did not have appendicitis. She then became more unwell on her way home and represented where she was found to have a perforated appendix.
- Option 3 – She was kept in hospital for two days then finally had an ultrasound/CT scan which showed she did not have appendicitis and was discharged.

**INTRODUCTION AND HISTORY**

- Confirm patient details
- History – ensure you ask about SOCRATES for abdominal pain
- Examination – Ask for observations, abdominal examination, speculum, bimanual examination
- Investigations – Bloods (FBC, U&Es, LFTs, CRP, group and save), venous blood gas for lactate, ECG for tachycardia, urine dipstick and pregnancy test, USS abdomen

**MANAGEMENT**

- Explain that you think most likely diagnosis is appendicitis and you will organise an USS abdomen to look for signs of this.
- In the interim, you will admit her and start her on intravenous antibiotics.

**TO THROW YOU OFF**

- Patient has been waiting in A and E for a few hours – so start off by apologising
- Patient states they are unable to stay in hospital.
- Listen and explore concerns – works as a lawyer and has urgent deadlines and childcare issues.
- Empathise, but explain why you would recommend admission – If appendicitis and not treated, can worsen and cause severe infection which can be potentially life threatening. If appendicitis, may need surgical management

**DEALING WITH ANGRY PATIENT**

- Listen
- Apologise
- If appropriate, explain that you will put in an incident form, speak to seniors and provide feedback to the staff involved. Consider organising teaching on appendicitis. Give her the option of PALS.
- Find out how she is recovering post-operatively and if she has any questions about appendicitis and post-op management.

# DEALING WITH AN ANGRY PATIENT

**APOLOGISE**

- Listen, allow patient time to express their concerns
- Apologise for the distress caused

**INVESTIGATE**

- Speak to your senior, obtain notes and establish how care could have been improved
- You will put in an incident report, which goes to the management team and senior doctors who will investigate the case
- You can organise teaching to raise awareness or bring up the problem at weekly teaching to bring about awareness and prevent recurrence
- Patient can also put in direct complaint through PALS which will again be investigated through similar pathways.

**FOLLOW UP**

- Organise meeting in 2 weeks and we can keep you informed about what we have found and changes we are making
- If you want you can arrange for a senior to speak to them sooner?
- Is there anything else that we can do to help you?

**GENERAL MEDICAL CARE**

- How are they otherwise? How is their recovery and symptoms
- If complaint is about lack of explanation regarding condition and management, explain again and provide leaflet.

# PRE-OPERATIVE ASSESSMENT

You are reviewing a 48 year old lady on the morning of her hysterectomy. She is having a hysterectomy for menorrhagia. As part of her routine pre-op review she has had a chest x-ray.

Chest X-ray: "Left sided lung nodule, suspicious of malignancy. CT scan recommended"

You have discussed with your consultant and anaesthetic colleagues and it is felt that her surgery needs to be delayed pending further investigation

**PART 2 OF STATION -**

The patient has returned a few weeks later after been advised that the CT is normal. She is upset about the cancer scare and for her operation being cancelled.

| | |
|---|---|
| HISTORY | • Introduce yourself to the patient<br>• Confirm patient details<br>• Confirm reasoning for the hysterectomy<br>• Ask about other medical conditions, drug history, family history, surgical history, social history (including smoking and occupation)<br>• Ask about symptoms – chest pain, shortness of breath, cough, haemoptysis, weight loss, fevers. |
| EXPLAINING PRE-OPERATIVE INVESTIGATION RESULTS | • Check understanding regarding pre-operative investigations<br>• Start with the "normal results" – e.g. normal blood count and heart trace<br>• Then explain that the chest x-ray showed some abnormal shadowing. "At this stage, we are unsure what the cause of the shadowing is. Sometimes, because a chest x-ray is a single image, there can be overlap of the structures in your chest and this can appear as shadowing, although it is in fact normal. However, there are other potential causes for this shadowing and the only way to distinguish is by doing further imaging"<br>• We will organise for you to have an urgent CT scan of the chest (a more specialised x-ray). This should happen within the next two weeks and we will review you with the results.""<br>• "Unfortunately, as we do not know what the cause of the shadowing is at this time, it would not be safe to put you through general anaesthesia and go ahead with the hysterectomy today. We will therefore have to book the hysterectomy at a later date depending on the results of these investigations." |
| DEALING WITH PATIENT'S CONCERNS | • The patient is very angry and states that she has been waiting for this operation for six months. She has told her relatives, organised child care and taken time off work. She states that her boss is going to be furious if she needs another 2 weeks off<br>• "I'm really sorry that you have to go through this. Is there anything we can do to help? If you want we can speak to someone at your workplace to explain the situation"<br>• The patient asks, "What could the other causes for this shadowing be?"<br>• There are lots of potential causes. These include chest infections, fluid around the heart or in the lungs, enlargement of the large blood vessel leaving the heart, or any kind of tumour in the lungs" |

## PART 2 OF STATION – DEALING WITH AN ANGRY PATIENT

- Listen. Apologise.
- "I'm sorry you were made to feel like you had cancer. Although it is one of the causes for shadowing, shadowing can be normal or due to other causes."
- "I will speak to my senior about your concerns, and we will review the notes and see what could have been done differently to improve your care and the way we communicated the results to you. I will also give some teaching to our team about shadowing on chest x-rays and how best to manage and communicate these to patients. If you wish to make a formal complaint, I can give you details of the PALS team who will escalate your concerns to senior medical staff who will again look into it."
- "In regards to the cancelled operation, when someone has shadowing on the lungs on a chest x-ray, we do not know if its normal or something more serious until they've had further investigations. At that point, it is unsafe to put someone through general anaesthesia without fully investigating it.
- "However, in your case the CT chest has come back normal, which is great news. I am going to call the booking team now and see when is the soonest that we can rearrange your operation. I will also inform my consultant and let them know about your results."
- "If you would benefit from speaking to one of my consultants now, I could arrange that for you. "

# BREAKING BAD NEWS: MISCARRIAGE

**THE BRIEF**

- A 32 year old lady has been having vaginal bleeding and abdominal cramping for the last few days.
- She has just had a pelvis ultrasound scan which shows a missed miscarriage at 6 weeks.
- Please see the patient and explain the ultrasound results.

# HOW TO MANAGE

| | |
|---|---|
| Introduction and history | • Introduce yourself & your role<br>• Make sure she is stable enough for a discussion (i.e. observation stable).<br>• Set the scene (go to a quiet room, switch off your bleep).<br>• Ask the patient if there is anyone she would like to call.<br>• Take a quick history (SOCRATES for pain, volume of bleeding, dizziness, shoulder tip pain, obstetric and gynaecological history including last menstrual period and outcome of any previous pregnancies, last smear test, history of sexually transmitted infections, any other medical/surgical/drug history or allergies. |
| Breaking Bad News | • Ascertain prior knowledge (what does she already know?)<br>• Give warning shots ("I am afraid it is not good news")<br>• Explain the ultrasound report:<br>  • Be clear ("You have had a miscarriage")<br>  • Don't waffle<br>  • No jargon<br>  • Don't give false hope<br>• Pause! Allow her the opportunity to cry and provide her tissues if she does.<br>• Be sympathetic but professional. |
| Further Information | • Once she has calmed down, give her some statistics:<br>  • It is NOT HER FAULT!<br>  • Miscarriages are very common (1 in 4).<br>  • Most miscarriages are one off (sporadic).<br>  • Chances of a future healthy pregnancy is the same as someone who has not had a miscarriage.<br>  • Most common cause is chromosomal abnormality in the fetus. No investigation unless three consecutive miscarriages.<br>  • No treatment to prevent miscarriage.<br>• Further management:<br>  • If the miscarriage is complete- no further treatment.<br>  • If the miscarriage is incomplete- give her further management options. |

# HOW TO MANAGE

**Further management options**

1) Letting nature take its course (expectant management)
    - Successful in 50% of women.
    - Bleeding and cramping can last up to 3 weeks.
    - If severe bleeding and pain, may need emergency admission.
2) Taking tablets (medical management)
    - Successful in 85% of women.
    - Medication allows neck of the womb to open and pregnancy tissue to pass.
    - Usually takes hours to days to work during which she can experience pain and heavy bleeding. Pain relief and anti-sickness tablets will be provided.
    - Can go home after tablet administered. However, if heavy bleeding may need admission.
3) Having an operation (surgical management)
    - Successful in 95% of women.
    - Done under general anaesthesia.
    - The neck of the womb is gently opened and pregnancy tissue is removed using a suction device. The procedure is called Surgical Management of Miscarriage (SMM).
    - It is a commonly performed operation and generally safe. However there is a small risk of complications (bleeding, infection, incomplete procedure and need for further intervention, uterine perforation). The risk of uterine perforation (making a hole in the uterus) is 5 in a 1000 but if this occurs, there is a risk of damage to structures in the tummy including bowel, bladder, tubes that go to the bladder (ureters) and blood vessels. In the event that the uterus is perforated, laparoscopy (keyhole surgery) or laparotomy (cut in the tummy) may be needed to check for/repair any damage.
    - The risk of infection is the same for surgical and medical management.

**Ending the consultation**

- Check her understanding.
- Ask if she has any questions.
- Acknowledge that you have given her a lot of information.
- Ask if she wants to go and think about the options.
- Offer her a second appointment once she has made a decision.
- Offer leaflet.
- Seek medical advice urgently if heavy bleeding, pain not relieved with analgesia, offensive smelling vaginal discharge or flu-like symptoms such as shivers or raised temperature.

# CHLAMYDIA IN AN ANGRY PATIENT

**THE BRIEF**

- A 30 year old patient with a one week history of abnormal vaginal discharge was seen last week in clinic and has come back to find out the results of her triple swabs and ultrasound.
- The ultrasound is normal, however, the swabs show that the patient has chlamydia.
- The patient has being waiting for 30 minutes.
- Please see the patient and inform her of the results.

# HOW TO ANSWER

**Introduction and dealing with an angry patient**

- Read the brief carefully (you are 30 minutes late!)
- Don't be fooled - this scenario is also a breaking bad news station.
- Introduce yourself and your role.
- Be prepared, the patient will be ANGRY!
- Listen to her and don't interrupt!
- APOLOGISE PROFUSELY!
- Explain to her that you were late because you were attending to another emergency.
- Offer her discussion with a more senior doctor.
- Offer her the contact details for Patient Advice and Liaison Service (PALS) if she remains angry.
- Never raise your voice.
- Remain calm, apologetic and sympathetic.

**Breaking Bad News**

- Recap, "I understand you've being having some discharge and had an ultrasound and some swabs taken. How are you feeling now?"
- Give the good news first, the ultrasound is NORMAL.
- "But I am afraid the swab results show you have chlamydia."
- Pause!
- "However, it is easily treated with antibiotics."
- Take a quick history, including sexual partners

**Further Information**

- Give her some information, SLOWLY, don't regurgitate everything you know. Avoid jargon.
  - Chlamydia is a sexually transmitted infection.
  - It is common amongst young people.
  - It is easily treated with oral antibiotics.
  - You can catch chlamydia when you have unprotected sex with someone who already has the infection. This can be by vaginal sex, oral sex or anal sex.

# HOW TO ANSWER

| | |
|---|---|
| Long term complications and further management | • Tell her about future complications<br>  • Chlamydia is unlikely to lead to any long-term problems if it is treated quickly. However, without treatment chlamydia can cause serious problems.<br>  • Women can develop pelvic inflammatory disease (PID). This can cause abdominal and pelvic pain. It can also lead to sub-fertility(difficulty getting pregnant) and ectopic pregnancy (a pregnancy that occurs outside the womb).<br>  • In rare cases, chlamydia may cause other symptoms such as arthritis (swollen joints) and inflammation of the eyes. (This is known as Reiter's syndrome and is more common in men).<br>• Further advice<br>  • "You should avoid any sex, even with a condom, until after both you and your partner have finished your treatment."<br>  • "You need to ensure you are tested to ensure the infection has gone after you complete treatment. You can do this at any sexual health clinic, and I can provide you with details of these."<br>  • "If you have chlamydia, you should also be tested for other sexually transmitted infections such as HIV, syphilis, hepatitis B and gonorrhoea, as you can have more than one infection at the same time."<br>  • Know the importance of **contact tracing**! "It is essential that your current sexual partner, and any other sexual partner you have had over the last six months, are tested and treated. This is to stop you getting the infection again, and also to prevent your partners developing any complications." |
| Ending the consultation | • Offer to answer any question she may have.<br>• Give an imaginary leaflet!<br>• Apologise again for being late! |

# DEEP VEIN THROMBOSIS IN A 15 YEAR OLD

**THE BRIEF**

- You have admitted a 15 year old girl to the hospital with a diagnosis of deep vein thrombosis. She started taking the oral contraceptive pill 6 months ago, which was prescribed by the GP.
- She is an occasional smoker. She has no past medical history. She currently had a boyfriend with whom she is sexually active. She has given you permission to discuss any details of her condition with her parents, but warns you that her father is "very old fashioned" and is not aware that she is on the pill or that she is sexually active.
- Please speak to her parents.

# HOW TO ANSWER

**Introduction**

- Introduce yourself and your role
- Check understanding (how much does the father know?)
- Reassure the father that his daughter is clinically stable.
- Give warning shots! "There are a few different issues that I need to discuss with you, some of which might come as a surprise to you."

**Clinical Explanation**

- Explain DVT in simple terminology
  - "Blood clot in the leg, restricting blood flow."
- Explain immediate treatment
  - "We have started your daughter on an injection that thins the blood. This will prevent more blood clots from forming."
- Explain long term management
  - "We will also need to start your daughter on another type of medication called warfarin. This will also work by thinning the blood and she will need to remain on it for at least 3 months. She will need regular monitoring of her blood clotting ability during this period."
- Explain any complications
  - "At the moment, things are under control, but if the blood clot dislodges it can travel to her lungs and cause problems with her breathing which can be serious."
- Do not overstate danger!
- "Long term problems are unlikely. However your daughter will be considered high risk for blood clots and hence in the future she may need to take precautions when taking long haul flights or deciding to get pregnant."

# HOW TO ANSWER

| | |
|---|---|
| Reasoning for PE | • "Why did this happen?"<br>  • Explain the risk factors for deep vein thrombosis.<br>  • "The majority of blood clots happen for no reason, but there are few things that make it more likely for someone to develop blood clots, for example taking the oral contraceptive pill or smoking."<br>  • If asked, state that the patient had two risk factors, oral contraceptive pill and smoking.<br>• Patient's father may become angry, in which case:<br>  • Apologise and acknowledge.<br>  • " I understand that some of this information may come as a surprise to you, I am sorry if that makes you feel upset."<br>• He may ask who started the contraceptive pill and how it was possible to without his consent:<br>  • Inform him that it was started by the GP.<br>  • Explain about Gillick competence.<br>  • "It is legal for doctors to prescribe medication for underage patients if they are able to understand the implications and effects of the medications."<br>  • "This is also done because it is preferable for teenagers to be using birth control and protection than having unprotected sexual intercourse because of fear that the information will be revealed to their parents." |
| Angry patient and completing the consultation | • The patient's father remains angry and wants to complain:<br>  • Apologise and remain calm.<br>  • Acknowledge it is a lot of information to take in.<br>  • Give him the opportunity to speak to a senior member of staff.<br>  • Give information about PALS (Patient Advice and Liaison Service).<br>  • Give him a leaflet on deep vein thrombosis. |

# COMMUNICATION STATION 1

## INSTRUCTIONS BEFORE ENTERING

You are the Senior House Officer in Accident and Emergency. Your next patient has been waiting a long time to see you. She has presented with chest pain. Please take a history, ask for relevant examination and investigation findings, and explain the diagnosis and treatment to the patient. You will be stopped at half time.

## HISTORY

You are a 23 year old female who has had sharp pain under her left breast since yesterday evening. Paracetamol does not relieve the pain. The pain is worse on taking a deep breath in. You have coughed up some fresh blood this morning. You are a smoker and are on the oral contraceptive pill (do not state unless specifically asked). You have never had a pulmonary embolism or deep vein thrombosis before. Your mum had a 'blood clot in her lungs'. You are not pregnant. No recent travel/surgery/fracture.

## EXAMINATION

- Chest – clear
- Heart sounds – normal
- Respiratory rate – 32
- Heart rate – 120
- Oxygen saturations – 96% on air
- Temperature – 37.0
- Left calf – red and painful

## INVESTIGATIONS

- Chest x-ray – normal
- Electrocardiogram – sinus tachycardia
- Troponin – negative
- D-dimer – positive
- Arterial blood gas – signs of respiratory alkalosis with mild hypoxia
- CT pulmonary angiogram – shows pulmonary embolism

## SECOND HALF OF SCENARIO

Stop candidate. Scenario moves forward 3 days. Patient has been admitted to hospital for treatment of her pulmonary embolism. She has now written a formal letter of complaint as she feels that there has been poor communication with her.

# COMMUNICATION STATION 1 - MARK SCHEME

| | |
|---|---|
| Introduces self, grade | /2 |
| Listens to patient ideas, concerns and expectations | /2 |
| History taking<br>• History of presenting complaint including assessment of pain and associated symptoms (shortness of breath, cough, calf pain)<br>• Risk factors for thromboembolic disease | /4 |
| Examination<br>• Observations<br>• Chest exam<br>• Leg exam | /3 |
| Investigations<br>• Chest X-ray<br>• Bloods including D-dimer<br>• Electrocardiogram (ECG)<br>• CT Pulmonary Angiogram (CTPA)/Ventilation Perfusion Scan (V/Q) | /3 |
| Management<br>• Offers analgesia and oxygen<br>• Treatment dose low molecular weight heparin pending investigations<br>• Need for warfarin for at least 3 months | /3 |
| Breaking bad news<br>• Asks patient what she knows<br>• Breaks news gently<br>• Explains diagnosis in simple terms | /2 |
| Managing an angry patient and complaint<br>• Listens to and empathises with patient's concerns<br>• Apologises to patient<br>• Explores events with patient<br>• Offers patient opportunity to talk to a senior<br>• Offers patient contact details of PALS if she wishes to take this further | /4 |
| Patient score | /3 |
| Examiner score | /4 |
| **Overall score** | **/30** |
| Feedback | |

# COMMUNICATION STATION 2

**INSTRUCTIONS BEFORE ENTERING**

You are the Senior House Officer in Accident and Emergency. Your next patient has presented with lower abdominal pain. Please take a brief history, ask for relevant examination and investigation findings, and explain the diagnosis to the patient. You will be stopped at half time.

**HISTORY**

You are a 19 year old female who has a history of lower abdominal pain and deep dyspareunia. This has been ongoing for two months, but has become unbearable over the past 24 hours. You have purulent vaginal discharge but no nausea or vomiting. You have no urinary or bowel symptoms. You broke up with your long term partner three months ago, and have had unprotected sexual intercourse with a new partner since then. Your periods are irregular and your last period was 3 weeks ago. You have never been pregnant.

**EXAMINATION**

- Chest – clear
- Heart sounds – normal
- Abdomen – diffuse lower abdominal tenderness
- Respiratory rate – 16
- Heart rate – 76
- Oxygen saturations – 100% on air
- Temperature – 38.5
- Pelvis – cervical excitation and bilateral adnexal tenderness

**INVESTIGATIONS**

- Urinary pregnancy test - negative
- Bloods – raised white cell count and C-reactive protein, otherwise normal
- Endocervical swab – chlamydia

**SECOND HALF OF SCENARIO**

Stop candidate. Scenario moves forward 4 weeks. The patient has returned to hospital. You are a different doctor. She is concerned that she believes the doctor she saw previously was rude, and led her to believe she will be infertile.

# COMMUNICATION STATION 2 - MARK SCHEME

| | |
|---|---|
| Introduces self, grade | /2 |
| Listens to patient ideas, concerns and expectations | /2 |
| History taking<br>• History of presenting complaint - including assessment of pain, discharge and deep dyspareunia<br>• Sexual history | /4 |
| Examination<br>• Observations<br>• Abdominal examination<br>• Pelvic examination | /3 |
| Investigations<br>• Urinary pregnancy test<br>• Full blood count, C-reactive protein<br>• Triple swabs | /3 |
| Management<br>• Assesses patient's current understanding<br>• Breaks news gently<br>• Explains diagnosis in simple terms<br>• Explains importance of contact tracing<br>• Explains importance of barrier contraception to reduce further risk<br>• Explain possible long term effects (subfertillty, ectopic pregnancy, chronic pain) | /3 |
| Managing an angry patient<br>• Listens to and empathises with patient's concerns<br>• Apologises to patient<br>• Explores events with patient<br>• Offers patient opportunity to talk to a senior<br>• Offers patient contact details of PALS if she wishes to take this further | /6 |
| Patient score | /3 |
| Examiner score | /4 |
| **Overall score** | **/30** |
| Feedback | |

# COMMUNICATION STATION 3

**INSTRUCTIONS BEFORE ENTERING:**
You are the Senior House Officer in A&E. Your next patient has presented with severe fatigue with a full blood count showing a haemoglobin of 62g/L. Please take a history, ask for relevant examination findings, and explain the diagnosis and treatment to the patient.

**HISTORY**
You are a 35 year old female who has been feeling tired all the time for the past few months. You have also been feeling short of breath on exertion. You have heavy periods, changing your pad up to every hour during the first few days, with clots and flooding. You have a thirty day regular cycle with seven days of bleeding. You use condoms for contraception, and do not think you could be pregnant. You have no other past medical history. Your smear tests are up to date and normal.

**EXAMINATION**
- Respiratory rate – 16
- Heart rate – 104
- Oxygen saturations – 99% on air
- Temperature – 37.2
- Chest – clear
- Heart sounds – normal
- Abdomen – soft but with a palpable fibroid uterus

# COMMUNICATION STATION 3 - MARK SCHEME

| | |
|---|---|
| Introduces self, grade | /2 |
| Listens to patient ideas, concerns and expectations | /2 |
| History taking<br>• Symptoms of anaemia<br>• History of menorrhagia (how heavy is the bleeding, need for double barrier protection, presence of clots, flooding)<br>• Menstrual history (regularity of cycle, how long bleeds last for, presence of inter-menstrual or post-coital bleeding)<br>• Gynaecological history (smear history, sexual history, contraception)<br>• Obstetric history (outcome of any pregnancies)<br>• Other potential causes of bleeding (haematemesis, malaena, night sweats, weight loss, swollen glands, recent surgery) | /4 |
| Examination<br>• Observations<br>• Abdominal examination | /3 |
| Management<br>• Discusses need for investigation of heavy menstrual bleeding with an ultrasound scan<br>• Discusses need for management of anaemia in the acute situation (see below) | /3 |
| Consent for a blood transfusion<br>• Explains reason for transfusion<br>• Explains benefits of a blood transfusion<br>• Explains risks of a blood transfusion (infection, allergic reaction, anaphylaxis, development of antibodies)<br>• Explains alternatives to blood transfusion (iron tablets and infusion)<br>• Explains what blood transfusion will involve (staying in hospital, cannula, close observation)<br>• Asks if patient has any questions<br>• Offers written information and time to make a decision | /6 |
| Patient score | /3 |
| Examiner score | /4 |
| **Overall score** | **/30** |
| Feedback | |

# COMMUNICATION STATION 4

**INSTRUCTIONS BEFORE ENTERING:**
You are the Senior House Officer in Gynaecology. Your next patient has presented with heavy vaginal bleeding. Please take a history, ask for relevant examination and investigation findings, and explain the diagnosis and treatment to the patient.

**HISTORY**
You are a 28 year old female with a 4 hour history of heavy vaginal bleeding and associated mild lower abdominal cramping pain. You are 10 weeks pregnant. You have been changing pads every 15-30 minutes and the bleeding is getting heavier. You are feeling very weak. You have had 1 previous termination of pregnancy and no previous sexually transmitted infections. You have not had an ultrasound in this pregnancy. You have no other past medical or surgical history.

**EXAMINATION**
- Respiratory rate – 20
- Heart rate – 120
- Blood Pressure – 90/60
- Oxygen saturations – 99% on air
- Temperature – 37.0
- Chest – clear
- Heart sounds – normal
- Abdominal exam – soft, non-tender
- Speculum – cervical os open with heavy vaginal bleeding

**INVESTIGATIONS**
- Urinary pregnancy test – positive
- Haemoglobin – 80g/L (previously 120g/L)

# COMMUNICATION STATION 4 - MARK SCHEME

| | |
|---|---|
| Introduces self, grade and role | /2 |
| Listens to patient ideas, concerns and expectations | /2 |
| History taking<br>• History of presenting complaint including assessment of severity of bleeding<br>• Symptoms of anaemia: dizziness/shortness of breath<br>• Risk factors for ectopic pregnancy (previous abdominal operations/ sexually transmitted infections, smoking, intrauterine coil devices) | /4 |
| Examination<br>• Observations<br>• Abdominal examination<br>• Pelvic examination | /2 |
| Investigations<br>• Haemoglobin<br>• Group and save/cross match<br>• Urinary pregnancy test | /2 |
| Management<br>• Resuscitate (cannula, intravenous fluids)<br>• Consider blood<br>• Senior support | /2 |
| Breaking bad news<br>• Explain to patient that she is miscarrying<br>• Breaks news gently<br>• Explains in simple terms | /3 |
| Consent for "Surgical Management of Miscarriage (SMM)"<br>• Explains what procedure is<br>• Explains reason for procedure<br>• Explains how the procedure is performed<br>• Explains risks of procedure<br>    • General (bleeding and need for blood transfusion, infection, pain, thromboembolic disease)<br>    • Specific (uterine perforation and damage to nearby structures which could require laparoscopy/laparotomy and repair of damage, incomplete procedure and need for repeat procedure)<br>• Asks if patient has any questions | /6 |
| Patient score | /3 |
| Examiner score | /4 |
| **Overall score** | **/30** |
| Feedback | |

# COMMUNICATION STATION 5

**INSTRUCTIONS BEFORE ENTERING:**
You are the Senior House Officer in Gynaecology. You are seeing patients pre-operatively. Your next patient is Mrs Brown. Mrs Brown is a 48 year old lady who is due to have a hysterectomy today due to long standing menorrhagia resistant to conservative measures. Her pre-operative assessment included a chest x-ray which is reported as, "Left sided lung nodule, suspicious of malignancy. CT scan recommended". You have discussed with your consultant and anaesthetic colleagues and it is felt that her surgery needs to be delayed pending further investigations.

**HISTORY**
You are a 48 year old lady with a longstanding history of menorrhagia. You have tried numerous treatment options in the past without any success and therefore a hysterectomy was organised. You have been waited for this hysterectomy for six months and have made numerous arrangements. You work as a lawyer and have arranged for other lawyers to cover your cases whilst you have the operation and are recovering. You also have two children and your mum has travelled from Spain to help look after you and your children.

You have no history of chest pain/shortness of breath/cough/ haemoptysis/weight loss.

You are very upset that your hysterectomy is being delayed as you put a lot of work into organising childcare and rearranging your work schedule and are concerned about having to do this again when the operation is rearranged. You are also concerned regarding what the chest x-ray findings could indicate and if this could be cancerous.

**SECOND HALF OF SCENARIO**
Stop candidate.
"The scenario has moved forward 3 weeks. The patient has returned to hospital and has asked to speak to a doctor regarding a complaint. You are a different doctor. "

Patient: You have had your CT chest which was normal and therefore your operation was unnecessarily delayed. You feel that you were mislead into thinking you had cancer and have therefore been really stressed and upset the last few weeks.

# COMMUNICATION STATION 5 - MARK SCHEME

| | |
|---|---|
| Introduces self, grade and role | /1 |
| Confirms patients name and date of birth | /1 |
| Checks patients understanding (reason for hysterectomy/results of pre-operative investigations) | /2 |
| History taking<br>• Past Medical History<br>• Drug History<br>• Family History<br>• Social History (including smoking and occupation) | /3 |
| Symptoms related to chest x-ray findings<br>• Chest pain, shortness of breath, cough, haemoptysis, weight loss, fever, night sweats | /3 |
| Breaking bad news<br>• Explains chest x-ray findings in a sensitive manner<br>• Breaks news gently<br>• Explains in simple terms<br>• Explains that hysterectomy will need to be delayed pending further investigations<br>• Explain further investigations (CT scan) and follow up | /6 |
| Deals effectively with patients concerns and questions | /2 |
| Dealing with angry patient<br>• Listens to patient's concern<br>• Apologises to patient<br>• Explores events with patient<br>• Empathises with concerns<br>• Offers patient opportunity to talk to a senior<br>• Offers patient opportunity to make formal complaint with PALS | /5 |
| Patient score | /3 |
| Examiner score | /4 |
| **Overall score** | **/30** |
| **Feedback** | |

# COMMUNICATION STATION 6

**INSTRUCTIONS BEFORE ENTERING:**
You are an FY2 reviewing Miss Ramone in A and E. Miss Ramone is a 28 year old female who have come in with lower abdominal pain. Please take a history, ask for relevant examination and investigation findings, and explain the diagnosis and treatment to the patient.

**PATIENT'S HISTORY**
You are a 28 year old lady with a one day history of central to right iliac fossa pain. The pain has been constant and worsening despite taking co-codamol prior to attending hospital. You also have had loss of appetite, and have vomited once today. Severity of the pain is now 7/10.

You are G0P0, having had no previous pregnancies. You are sexually active with a regular partner and use condoms for contraception. You have never had any sexually transmitted infections. You have regular menstrual cycles occurring every 28 days lasting 5 days, with no menorrhagia, dysmenorrhoea, intermenstrual or post coital bleeding. Your smear tests are up to date and normal. Your last menstrual period was 3 weeks ago.

You have no past medical or surgical history of note. You are not on any medication and have no allergies. You are a non-smoker, drink alcohol socially and work as a lawyer.

When given the diagnosis of appendicitis and explained that you need to be admitted, you are not happy as you do not have childcare organised and have an important court case tomorrow that you cannot miss.

**EXAMINATION AND INVESTIGATION FINDINGS**
Observations – temperature 37.9 degrees, heart rate 89, blood pressure 120/80, respiratory rate 16, oxygen saturations 100% on air

Abdominal examination – Tender at McBurneys point with positive Rovsings sign. No guarding or rebound.

Speculum examination – Normal vagina, vulva and cervix. No adnexal or cervical tenderness.

Urinalysis – Urine dipstick NAD, urine pregnancy test negative.
Blood tests – WCC 16, CRP 100, Haemoglobin 120g/L, Lactate 1

**SECOND HALF OF SCENARIO**
Stop candidate.

"The scenario has moved forward 4 weeks. The patient has returned to hospital and has asked to speak to a doctor regarding a complaint. You are a different doctor. "

Patient: You spent two days waiting in hospital for an ultrasound scan which showed you did not have appendicitis and were then discharged. You therefore spent two days unnecessarily in hospital and missed an important court case. You are very angry and upset about this and the level of care in the hospital.

# COMMUNICATION STATION 6 - MARK SCHEME

| | |
|---|---|
| Introduces self, grade and role | /1 |
| Confirms patients name and date of birth | /1 |
| History taking<br>• Presenting Complaint<br>• Past Medical History<br>• Past Obstetric/Gynaecology History<br>• Drug History<br>• Family History<br>• Social History (including smoking and occupation) | /5 |
| Examination and Investigations<br>• Observations<br>• Abdominal examination<br>• Speculum examination and vaginal examination<br>• Urine dipstick and urinary pregnancy test<br>• Blood tests – FBC, U&E, CRP, Group and Save, venous blood gas<br>• Ultrasound/CT scan | /5 |
| Counselling and Management<br>• Offer analgesia<br>• Explains likely diagnosis of appendicitis and need for admission and potential surgery (depending on senior review and imaging)<br>• Nil by mouth | /4 |
| Deals effectively with patients concerns and questions | /2 |
| Dealing with angry patient<br>• Listens to patient's concern<br>• Apologises to patient<br>• Explores events with patient<br>• Empathises with concerns<br>• Offers patient opportunity to talk to a senior<br>• Offers patient opportunity to make formal complaint with PALS | /5 |
| Patient score | /3 |
| Examiner score | /4 |
| **Overall score** | **/30** |
| **Feedback** | |

# COMMUNICATION STATION 7

**INSTRUCTIONS BEFORE ENTERING:**
You are the FY2 in the General Surgery clinic today - your consultant has been called away to an emergency in A&E. The clinic is running 1 hour late.

Your next patient is 30 year old Mr Smith, who had an emergency appendectomy 6 months ago. He had presented to A&E with RIF pain and vomiting, and had surgery the next morning. He was meant to be followed up in clinic 12 weeks later but an appointment had unfortunately not been made for him. He has not been updated on the histology results.

Appendix tissue: normal tissue, no signs of inflammation. Please inform the patient about the histology results.

**PATIENT HISTORY**
You came to A&E 6 months ago with a 1 day history of right sided abdominal pain - despite antibiotics and painkillers you were not feeling well. You were consented for an appendicectomy but on the day of the surgery you wanted to speak to a doctor again about whether this surgery was necessary, but were not given the opportunity to do so.

You are extremely upset and angry about having waited 1 hour for your clinic appointment - this has made you late for work. You are also upset that they had not made a follow up appointment for you 12 weeks after surgery, and that you have waited 6 months to see them.

When informed that your histology results were normal, you became even more upset as you are now confident the surgery was unnecessary and that it cost you a lot of money as you are a self-employed contractor and had to take time off work.

*Decline a full history and examination

## SECOND HALF OF THE SCENARIO
Stop candidate.

"Mr Smith has returned to your clinic 3 months later - he has written a letter to yourself and the consultant:

I want to apologise for my behaviour in my last clinic appointment. Due to my frustrations, I behaved poorly towards the doctor.

He wants to speak to you to apologise to you."

Patient: After having had time to calm down, you would like to apologise to the doctor for your earlier behaviour.

# COMMUNICATION STATION 7 - MARK SCHEME

| | |
|---|---|
| Introduces self, grade and role | /1 |
| Confirms patients name and date of birth | /1 |
| Apologises firstly for the delay in reviewing the patient today, and for missed follow up appointment | /2 |
| Checks patients understanding of reason for appendicectomy, and briefly cover symptoms leading up to it. Can offer to examine and take a history but does not persist with this line of questions once patient declines. | /4 |
| Explains histology findings in simple terms | /4 |
| Deals effectively with patients concerns and questions | /2 |
| Dealing with angry patient<br>• Listens to patients concern<br>• Apologises to patient for lack of review before theatre<br>• Able to placate patient when he feels surgery was useless (in light of normal histology)<br>• Explores events and empathises with concerns<br>• Acknowledge issues raised and offers formal complaint with PALS<br>• Offer patient an opportunity to talk to senior<br>• Offer to write letter for employers regarding delay in appointment | /5 |
| Second half of station:<br>Ask patient how he is now<br>Able to keep conversation going<br>Offers to answer any further questions | /5 |
| Patient score | /3 |
| Examiner score | /4 |
| **Overall score** | **/30** |
| **Feedback** | |

Printed in Great Britain
by Amazon

41519952R00071